HOMESTEADING

What Things You Can Do With Your Self Sufficient Homestead For Raising Livestock

(Easy Homemade Insecticides And Traps)

Roger Fincher

Published by John Kembrey

Roger Fincher

All Rights Reserved

Homesteading: What Things You Can Do With Your Self Sufficient Homestead For Raising Livestock (Easy Homemade Insecticides And Traps)

ISBN 978-1-77485-129-6

All rights reserved. No part of this guide may be reproduced in any form without permission in writing from the publisher except in the case of brief quotations embodied in critical articles or reviews.

Legal & Disclaimer

The information contained in this book is not designed to replace or take the place of any form of medicine or professional medical advice. The information in this book has been provided for educational and entertainment purposes only.

The information contained in this book has been compiled from sources deemed reliable, and it is accurate to the best of the Author's knowledge; however, the Author cannot guarantee its accuracy and validity and cannot be held liable for any errors or omissions. Changes are periodically made to this book. You must consult your doctor or get professional medical advice before using any of the suggested remedies, techniques, or information in this book.

Upon using the information contained in this book, you agree to hold harmless the Author from and against any damages, costs, and expenses, including any legal fees potentially resulting from the application of any of the information provided by this guide. This disclaimer applies to any damages or injury caused by the use and application, whether directly or indirectly, of any advice or information presented, whether for breach of contract, tort, negligence, personal injury, criminal intent, or under any other cause of action.

You agree to accept all risks of using the information presented inside this book. You need to consult a professional medical practitioner in order to ensure you are both able and healthy enough to participate in this program.

Table of Contents

INTRODUCTION 1

CHAPTER 1: WHY HOMESTEADING IS A GOOD DECISION .. 3

CHAPTER 2: EXTENDING THE GARDENING SEASON 22

CHAPTER 3: PRESERVE YOUR FOOD FOR FUTURE USES ... 33

CHAPTER 4: HOMESTEAD PROJECTS 39

CHAPTER 5: TESTING AND PREPARATION OF SOIL TYPES 48

CHAPTER 6: ORGANIC PRODUCTION 56

CHAPTER 7: LET'S START! THE BASIC STEPS TO GROWING IN CONTAINERS 77

CHAPTER 8: PLANT NUTRITION & TROUBLESHOOTING ... 88

CHAPTER 9: CHOOSING THE IDEAL PLANTS FOR YOUR GARDEN 123

CHAPTER 10: 7 REASONS WHY YOU SHOULD GET GROW YOUR OWN VEGETABLES 144

CHAPTER 11: HOW TO MAKE YOUR OWN ENERGY 148

CHAPTER 12: THE BEST TYPES OF FRUITS FOR HOME GARDENING 152

CHAPTER 13: MAXIMIZING YOUR SPACE 165

CHAPTER 14: THE NEED FOR COMMUNITY 167

CHAPTER 15: HOW TO BUILD A NEW FLOWER BED FOR ALL YOUR FAVORITE BLOOMS 171

CHAPTER 16: HOW TO LEARN ABOUT HOMESTEADING: 188

CHAPTER 17: SAVE AND GENERATE YOUR OWN ENERGY 199

CONCLUSION 201

Introduction

This book provides proven strategies and steps on how to homesteal your own land and reduce your costs by using your backyard farm. There are many ways to homestead in modern times. Homesteading's main purpose is to help you become self-sufficient and reduce your dependence on others.

This book will answer all your questions about homesteading, and how to build your farm from the extra space in your backyard. You will reap more benefits in both monetary and non-monetary terms by using the extra space you have.

This book introduces homesteading and will help you understand how to reduce your expenses so that you can live a sustainable life. This book also includes several methods for homesteading.

Homesteading can be done in many ways. However, it is important to plan your backyard farm properly. To help you make the perfect plan, I have included all the necessary rules. This book also includes the methods that you can transform your backyard into a four-season farm. This book is an essential guide for anyone who wants to homestead and learn from the basics.

Thank you again for downloading the book. I hope that it was enjoyable!

Chapter 1: Why Homesteading Is A Good Decision

Comprehensively characterized, Home steading is a way of life of independence and it is portrayed by means horticulture and it's a family unit compound for a solitary more distant family.

A portion of the advantages that we get when we pick homesteading are -
Quality of food and life: Regardless of the reasons homesteaders accommodate carrying on with an existence of independence, by the day's end, nature of food and personal satisfaction is the primary reasons why they picked thusly of life. Natively constructed yogurt and eggs have a taste that leaves your mouth salivating for additional. Hand crafted bread is so delicate and new that the locally acquired new appears to be bland

in correlation. Great quality food causes us for a superior way of life.

Happy and Healthy Life: There is various medical advantages related with homesteading. The food you produce, without a doubt, has various medical advantages than mass-delivered nourishments. Eggs, bread, meat and other natively constructed nourishments have their supplements unblemished while mass-created food things will in general miss out on fundamental supplements as they sit in the case sitting tight for you in the grocery store. In addition, your lawn chicks and goats will in general devour an assortment of sound nourishments that causes them produce supplement rich food.

In expansion to being supplement rich, local products of the soil don't have unsafe pesticides and synthetic concoctions in them. Since local food are not hereditarily altered or falsely aged, they hold their normal shading, taste and supplements. Various ailments that outcome from manufacturing plant cultivating, for example, E.coli, salmonella and different infections are wiped out in local nourishments.

The medical advantages of homesteading are not restricted to food; truth be told, the measure of activity you get additionally encourages you have a sound existence. The measure of work engaged with homesteading is especially usefully to your body. Regardless of whether you are into metropolitan homesteading, you get a ton of physical exercise which is incredible for your wellbeing and general prosperity.

Economically Beneficial: Baking your own bread is route less expensive than purchasing a portion of bread from the close by grocery store. A few people may disclose to you that homesteading includes putting resources into a great deal of extravagant devices and devices; in any case, this is totally false. Making your own cleanser, bread, eggs, meat and bread goes far in helping you set aside a great deal of cash. Actually, homesteading likewise includes different methods of safeguarding food things in an earth cordial way.

You can undoubtedly grow a compartment garden utilizing save holders at home or likewise search for square foot cultivating strategies.

Environmental Friendly: Our innovation enhanced way of life has been reliably burdening our planet's assets so much that we are very nearly depleting various non-inexhaustible assets. A large portion of us accept that on the off chance that we move from heading out in vehicles to going openly transport or going in for carpooling, you are sparing the planet. The facts confirm that carpooling and going in open transportation helps spare gallons of oil, we ought to likewise comprehend that it isn't sufficient to help spare the planet. Shipping organic products, vegetables and other food items from the ranch to our home expends several gallons of oil. Homesteading and cultivating can help spare the planet in various different manners as well. Industrial facility cultivating and mass-assembling of items is expending a great deal of assets. Actually, the poisons from these ranches and production lines are gagging our regular water and soil assets. They are hurting the world's fix and reclamation endeavors. In any case, this doesn't imply that you need to surrender in absolute irritation and surrender trust in a superior future. You don't need to run off into a cavern or surrender your extravagant home in the city. Metropolitan homesteading causes you hold your home in the city and keep on improving your life and spare the earth too.

Creating a Sense of Togetherness: The possibility of independence and fellowship appear complete opposites and conflicting. Nonetheless, there are more identified with one another than we accept. At the point when you take up metropolitan homesteading, you are in a roundabout way promising others in your locale to hold turns in improving the world a much spot to live. You will be amazed to discover that various individuals would be more than ready to help you in your undertakings. Independence isn't tied in with giving just to self or confining from others. Indeed, metropolitan homesteading is being taken up as a network exertion in various spots.

Personally Gratifying: There is nothing all the more satisfying that seeing a wonderful pack of carrots or preparing a huge portion of bread — all by you. The feeling of fulfillment and pride you get by developing your own food, raising goats and chickens and making your own cleansers and different utilities can't be contrasted and getting them from the market. You accomplish a profound feeling of fulfillment, accomplishment, and furthermore build up a good and solid demeanor towards life.

One of the lesser referenced reasons homesteading is proceeding to develop in notoriety and the "prepper" development has grabbed hold is that of security of private property and the lives of families over the globe. Wrongdoing insights are not diminishing and the quantity of home intrusions is on the ascent in numerous bigger metropolitan zones. Recognizing this need, numerous states have sanctioned laws that permit people to secure themselves in their homes utilizing dangerous power when justified.

Presently we dive into an extremely dubious subject - that of security for your residence and the most ideal approach to ensure what is yours. We will begin with essential estate security - a couple of good judgment thoughts that will ideally guard your property and your families.

Hard-Wired Lighting. Contingent on the accessibility of power and the bounty in that, open air lighting can go about as a viable hindrance to wrongdoing. Lawbreakers like to prowl in obscurity, lights on around your residence makes an issue for them. Open air lighting used to be extremely costly too, notwithstanding, a unimaginable aspect concerning innovation is that today, even the low wattage bulbs produce a ton of light. Your power utilization may not be as awful as you may might suspect.

Solar Powered Motion Lights. The main cost you will have is that of procurement and establishment. Movement recognizing illuminating not just lights significant zones of your residence, the give the feeling that somebody is home and watching - regardless of whether you're most certainly not. One thing to note, nonetheless, is that utilization of movement identifying lighting is delivered ineffectual if it's introduced near your domesticated animal's zones. The development of your animals will have the lights flashing throughout the night.

Locks. Another thing from the "significant handle of the conspicuous record" no doubt, nonetheless, a basic lock can shield your estate from attack generally. Locking instruments, costly hardware and your home with the utilization of rock solid locks will, in any event, slow down the eventual criminal on the grounds that once in a while will the criminal component convey jolt cutters in their glove compartment. The dismal truth is that if a trouble maker is resolved to break into your home and take your property, there is almost no that can or will stop the person in question. The target with locks is to in any event baffle and moderate them down.

Firearms (home security). As questionable as it might be, there is nothing that will place the dread of the Almighty in the hearts and psyches of crooks than the sound of a siphon activity shotgun racking a shell. It is a generally realized sound that says, "In case you're willing to come here, be happy incredible what you're going to take."

Shotguns can take a touch of becoming acclimated to in light of the forceful backlash. Before a shotgun is utilized - just like the case with each gun, take it to the range and toss some lead and acclimate yourself with the vibe, the weight and the sound of the shotgun. [Note: Urban homesteaders should initially check with nearby specialists and realize what the necessities are for the ownership and utilization of guns. Each region is extraordinary, hence it's smarter to be sheltered than sorry later.

Predators. Coyotes, wildcats, and mountain lions can be considered "aggravation creatures." In numerous states, these disturbance creatures procure their title on account of the harm they do to animals. Prior to bringing down any predators, check with your state untamed life office and discover the guidelines in that since they differ incredibly from state to state, nation to nation.

A shotgun, likewise, is certainly not a decent gun to take these predators. A shotgun has an exceptionally short range and is incapable. Then again, a rifle with an economical extension, loaded with at any rate .223 round, will bring down a coyote, a catamount or even a mountain lion at 75 yards easily. Obviously, metropolitan homesteaders infrequently need to stress over such predators, neither will they have domesticated animals meandering around the back yard. There are, notwithstanding, non-deadly techniques for predator disposal. For instance, most predators, for example, wildcats and coyotes, are frightened of human fragrance. Drag your newly utilized shower towel around behind you as you hover the external limits of your property. For the genuinely daring and daring, human pee has a particular fragrance and endures well after the aroma gets imperceptible by the human olfactory sense.

Remember those solar powered motion-activated lights we discussed a few paragraphs ago? Those too can be used to deter predation to your livestock if installed at the perimeters of your livestock pens. This is not a long-term fix, because many predators will get used to that type of stimuli and not be effected by it at all. The best way to use these non-lethal means is to move them to different areas frequently so as to change how the predator sees or senses the deterrent.

Protecting your investment, your commitment to self-sufficiently sadly include the need to protect you and yours. It is truly unfortunate that the conversation must exist as to making a decision to use deadly force to protect you and yours. We live in trying times and as mentioned previously, one of the reasons so many people desire to live off the proverbial grid and become self-sufficient is because of the dangers lurking in every corner of the globe.

Urban Homesteading Vs. Rural Homesteading

Both metropolitan and country homesteading offers an incredible feeling of fulfillment of getting things done without anyone else. Developing foods grown from the ground in a lawn garden, cooking them, building furniture and instruments for our homes, and furthermore learning new strategies of independence and re-learning old and overlooked aptitudes is homesteading nowadays. Homesteading gives a great deal of autonomy and decisions. It shields us from obligation emergency, offers more decisions for seeking after diversions and interests, offers more prominent security in the hours of monetary lull and downturn, and shields us from ecological risks.

While homesteading hurls an image of living in the wide open with immense (read sections of land) regions of land standing by to be plowed and furrowed, it is simply only a daytime dream. Actually, country homesteading is conceivable just for individuals who have the advantage of land and time.

In the event that you are living in the city, homesteading may appear to be a removed unthinkable dream. Abandoning luxuries like mobile phone, web, home conveyance, trash pickup, power, gas, close by neighbors and simple transportation may appear to be a weighty cost to pay. Living in the wide open may be serene, quiet and more laid-back; in any case, this isn't for everybody.

Most manuals on homesteading will disclose to you that you need to surrender the extravagances of the city, gather your packs and settle down on a ranch to take up homesteading. Truth be told, many homesteading specialists likewise talk about planting and raising livestock on sections of land of land. The bounty and accessibility of land will before long become a weight when you don't have the foggiest idea how to manage it. Because you don't have a section of land of land to call your own, don't abandon homesteading. You can keep on remaining independent with metropolitan homesteading. Indeed, even with a solitary square foot of land in the city or an overhang to call your own, you can develop your preferred foods grown from the ground and live a solid life. On the off chance that you have the advantage of land some place in the open country, and are eager to surrender the delights of the city, you are free to attempt rustic homesteading. Be that as it may, if space is a requirement and you would prefer not to lose your city life, you can attempt metropolitan homesteading and appreciate similar advantages of provincial living.

Homesteading and Permaculture

Homesteading and permaculture are identified with each other; they proliferate the ideas of independence, care for the planet, individuals and returning normal assets to the planet. It is the idea of supportable technique for farming. Permaculture reasoning is working with nature and not neutralizing its standards. It is taking a gander at the scene of a spot, comprehend the elements of species and unite different pieces to make one better item. Permaculture diminishes squander, limit work and contribution of vitality into making items. It is tied in with bringing all the bits of an idea together so greatest advantages are benefited from it. Permaculture is an all-inclusive part of natural and ecological plan.

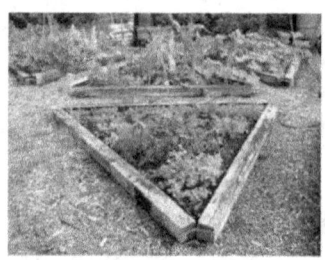

Nursery with Permaculture picture from Flickr via Sean

Homesteading - A social, economic and lifestyle choice
To totally comprehend the ideas of homesteading, you should initially comprehend its foundations and explanations behind its prevalence. In 1862, the U.S. government offered almost 160 sections of land of free land to individuals who vowed to live on it effectively for quite a long time. Numerous families had a special interest in this land

and began developing yields, raising creatures, developing area, and dealt with the family utilizing hand crafted things.

The Homestead Act of 1862 was viewed as an exertion by the legislature of U.S. to populate already undesired pieces of land. Countries that were occupied with country building, begun tempting individuals to populate and develop on these parcels and create self-food techniques. More Homestead acts were started in the late nineteenth and mid 20thcenturies to drive country fabricating and populating explicit regions of the country. A restored enthusiasm for homesteading began to be found in the 1930's and 1940's.

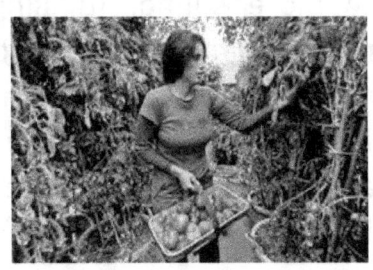

Making your own nursery makes a steady method of living picture from Flickr by Ian Livesey

Homesteading, notwithstanding being a social cycle of making independence, is a monetary decision to guarantee autonomy and confidence. Homesteading not just permits you to deliver food all alone, it additionally causes you sell your produce — food and different items — to others to help improve your monetary status.

Homesteading is a direction for living for some, and various individuals who are homesteading have communicated a profound feeling of fulfillment and happiness with their way of life and way of life. They feel that their lifestyle is unmistakably more sound, fulfilling and remunerating than the typical metropolitan lifestyles. Metropolitan Homesteading is definitely not a watered-down variant of rustic homesteading; actually, it is an undeniable idea that has various advantages.

Animals can be a staple of the homesteading way of life, giving a different wellspring of essential nurturing protein and assorted variety in supper readiness picture from Flickr by Ryan Li

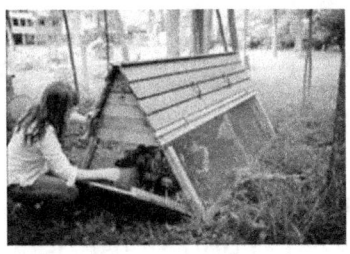

Chapter 2: Extending The Gardening Season

For some special gardeners, it's hard to imagine taking a season off from gardening. Luckily, there are many ways you can extend your gardening season:

Cold Frames: Cold frames are a wonderful way to extend your gardening season.Learn how to build your own cold frames in this post.

Hoop Houses: A hoop house is a way to extend your growing season if you have raised beds.

Build a Greenhouse: You can buy an already made greenhouse to garden all year round, or you can build your own.

Grow some plants indoors: I don't have luck with indoor plants. I have too much shade around my home, so I don't have enough sunlight for successful indoor Planting.

Harvest and preserving the Crops/Aftermath

Dehydrate your produce: Dehydrating is a great way to preserve excess fruits and vegetables from your garden. Make sure to get a good-quality dehydrator for the best success (like this one).

Start canning: Canning excess produce.

Use a Root Cellar: If you are lucky, you live somewhere where you can dig deep in your land and make your own root cellar (or maybe your home has a basement to use as a root cellar).

How to sustain your garden without need for resources like supplemental watering or potentially toxic inputs like pesticides and herbicides.

Use of Organic Methods

Mulching all uncovered soil for water retention, weed control, and to improve the soil's structure.Best are shredded hard wood or bark, bark chips, cocoa hulls or leaf mold (composted leaves).f more fertilizer is necessary, using organic sources only (e.g., compost tea or fish- or seaweed-based).

Choosing pest- and disease-resistant plants.For pests, using preventive practices first (like ensuring good air circulation) and taking action only when a plant is endangered.Then using the least invasive or toxic methods first, like horticultural oil for scale and mites, But for caterpillars, beetles and mosquitoes, baking soda for black spot and powdery mildew, and SAFER brand soap for many problem insects. For pests, using biological and physical barrier controls like bait traps, hard sprays of water to remove aphids, removal by hand, and diatomaceous earth for slugs.

Minimizing or avoiding the use of pesticides, herbicides, and synthetic fertilizers.If pesticides are used, starting with the least toxic, like insecticidal soap, and steering clear of broad spectrum insecticides.

Weeding by hand or using a 10 percent vinegar solution. In lawns, by using a high mower setting, applying an organic fertilizer in the fall, and applying lime, as needed. Always testing the soil before adding amendments like lime.

Water Quality and Conservation

1. Watering smart - directly to the root zone by hand or using soaker or drip irrigation, and preferably in the morning.Avoiding sprinklers. Watering according to plant needs, not a rigid schedule. Watering infrequently but deeply - no fine mists.

2. Grouping plants with similar water needs. Keeping rain on your property using rain garden techniques and rain barrels.(Rain gardens are depressions in the soil that are planted with water-loving plants.)

3.Stabilizing stream banks with the use water-loving plants that reduce soil erosion, like liriope.

4.Minimizing bare soil and stabilizing slopes by planting ground covers.

5.Replacing or eliminating lawns.

6. Minimizing the use of impervious surfaces so rainwater can be filtered before reaching the storm water system.

7. Keeping trash, yard waste, fertilizers and de-icers off paved surfaces.

8. Growing drought-tolerant plants.

9. Weeding regularly - because weeds compete for water with the plants you want.

10. letting lawns go dormant in the summer.

Sustaining Wildlife

Most discussions of sustainable gardening include a word about sustaining the world outside the confines of the garden itself, by providing for local wildlife and avoiding plants that will invade and harm nearby natural areas. So eco-friendly, sustainable gardeners are increasingly choosing plants that sustain insects, birds and other critters we love.Locally native plants, especially trees, are generally best at doing that.We're careful to avoid known invasive plants.And to provide for wildlife, we're willing to incorporate ponds and other water features in our gardens, even if they require a bit of extra maintenance.

Five intrinsic characteristics of home gardens:

1) Are located near the residence.
2) Contain a high diversity of plant.
3) Production is supplemental rather than a main source of family consumption and income.
4) Occupy a small area.
5) Are a production system that the poor can easily enter at some level.

The role of home gardens as agroforestry or food production systems, or a combination of both. Home gardens are ecologically divided into two categories: tropical and temperate. Much of the literature focuses on home gardens in the tropical areas in Central and South America. There is also a substantial interest for home gardens in South and South-East Asia and Africa. Conversely, only a few documented studies exist on home gardens from temperate regions and from developed countries.

Home gardens are commonly established on lands that are marginal or not suitable for field crops or forage cultivation because of their size, topography, or location. The specific size of a home garden varies from household to household and, normally, their average size is less than that of the arable land owned by the household. However, this may not hold true for those families that do not own agricultural land and for the landless. New innovations and techniques have made home gardening possible even for the families that have very little land or no land at all. The home gardens may be delimited by physical demarcations such as live fences or hedges, fences, ditches or boundaries established through mutual understanding. Application of kitchen waste, animal manure, and other organic residues has been a practice amongst home gardeners and this exercise has helped to considerably increase the productivity and fertility of these gardens.

The key characteristics of a typical home garden

While some similarities exist across the board, each home garden is unique in structure, functionality, composition, and appearance as they depend on the natural ecology of the location, available family resources such as labor, and the skills, preferences, and enthusiasm of family members. Home garden cultivation tends to be quite dynamic. The decisions related to the selection of crops, procuring inputs, harvesting, management, and so forth are mostly driven by the consumption and income generation needs of the household. A study from Indonesia observed that the structure, composition, intensity of cultivation, and diversity of home gardens can be subjected to the socioeconomic status of the household. For instance, as the families became economically stable their cultivation shifted from staples to horticultural crops and some families began to raise livestock. Differentiated two types of home gardens:

1) Subsistence gardens
2) Budget gardens.

Access to planting material and social capital are noted as important attributes to species diversity in gardens. Collectively, the ecological potential, economic status, and social elements influence the presence of food and non-food crops and animals in the garden. Additionally, limitations resulting from factors such opportunities for off-farm employment and family structure as well as local customs influence the development and composition of the gardens.

The home garden frequently uses family labor - women, children, and elders are of particular importance in their management but, depending on the economic capacity and affordability, households may hire wage laborers to cultivate and maintain the home garden that in turn affect the composition and intensity of home garden activities. Like any other food production system, home gardens may be vulnerable to harsh environmental conditions such as drought and floods. Despite the fact that home gardening activities demand a lesser amount of horticultural and agronomic know-how, crop losses and other negative implications can be reduced when the household members are empowered with better skills and knowledge .

Experiences of home gardens from developing countries

Home gardens have been an integral part of local food systems in developing countries around the world. Many studies provide descriptive evidence and analysis of home gardens in developing countries in Asia, Africa, and Latin America and pinpoint their numerous benefits to communities and families. They encapsulate perpetual small-scaled subsistence agricultural systems established by the households to obtain and supplement the food requirements of the family. Home gardens are mainly intended to grow and produce food items for family consumption, but they can be diversified to produce outputs that have multiple uses including indigenous medicine and home remedies for certain illnesses, kindling and alternative fuel source, manure, building material, and animal feed. Home gardening benefits is broadly categorized into three components: (1) social; (2) economic; and (3) environmental benefits. These benefits are presented and explained through the vast experiences on home gardens from developing nations around the world.

Chapter 3: Preserve Your Food For Future Uses

Try these simple methods to preserve your extra food for the future uses:

Freezing

In the old days, people were habitual to get ice from the neighboring mountain to preserve food. Now, you have electrical freezers to preserve your foods. These freezers can change the texture of the most vegetables and fruits, but the fish and meat will not change their texture. In the summer days, you can freeze your berries to make smoothies and bake cakes. It will be good to freeze fruits and vegetables in batches. For instance, you can spread out fresh berries or other fruits on a baking tray and place it in the freezer. Once they become solid, you can put them in a bag. This will avoid clumps of your fruits, because clumps are difficult to separate without a thawing process.

If you want to keep food fresh, you can prepare packages and freeze meats, soups, bread, fruits, casseroles, and cakes. You should freeze fresh food as quickly as possible to keep it at zero degrees. Packaging food in the freezer containers will avoid any deterioration. There is no need to open container in the freezer because the dry air of the freezer will deteriorate the food. There are a few things to avoid freezer burn:
• Reduce Exposure to Air: You should wrap the food tightly to avoid exposure to dry air.
• Avoid Fluctuating Temperature: It is essential to keep freezer close as much as you can, and try to determine the name of things that you want to remove from freezer, before opening it.
• Don't Overfill Freezer: There is no need to overly fill the freezer because it will

reduce the circulation of air and increase the speed of the damage.

Salting

Salting is a small category of the drying method. You can add salt in the products, such as fish and meat to extract moisture. This will reduce the bacterial content and make the food flexible for later use. Salt can make animal protein, a bit leathery.Beef jerky and salted cod are famous food items prepared with preserved meat.

Canning

If you want to can food, you have to heat food. This technique is developed by a French Chemist in 1795. This method was used to preserve food for Napoleon's army. It is a popular way to preserve fruits, meats, and vegetables. You can use both cans and glass jars to preserve food. It is important to sterilize these cans in boiling water along with lids for a few minutes. You can fill these cans and glass jars with jam, jelly or other content. Add brine or sugar syrup in the cans. After filling, you should keep the lid firmly, but don't make it too tight.

It is time to keep the jars in a pot with water, cover it and let it boil. You have to process if for almost ten minutes and now pull the jars or cans out from the hot water and let it cool. They will seal like a vacuum, once they cooled down. Cooking time will vary as per the requirements of each recipe.

Pickling

There is the main difference between canning and pickling that you will need salt and acid. You have to soak your produces in brine prepared with salt. Pickle them for the desired amount of time and transfer them in a jar full of vinegar. At this point, you can get the advantage of pickling method to vacuum seal your container. Pickling will not change the texture too much and the vegetables undergo a fermentation process. It can boost vitamin and level of Vitamin B6.

Drying

Drying is a great way to preserve fruits, herbs, vegetables, and meats. If you want to dry herbs, you can tie them together and hang in a sunny place. You have to dry moisture of food to protect it for a longer period of time. This practice is used throughout the world, such as southern Italy is famous to dry tomatoes and India is famous for drying mangoes and chilies. If you want to dry herbs, you can hang them in a sunny place away from moisture. You can dry fruits and vegetables, so place them on a clean surface, but select a sunny place to keep them in the sun for a few weeks. This method works the best in warm and dry climates. The electric dehydrating machine is a modern method to dry fruits and vegetables.

Salt Curing and Brining

It is an old method to preserve meat because the salt creates an inhospitable environment for bacteria and microorganism. You can rub the mixture of sugar and salt on the pieces of fresh meat, pack it tightly into a crock and store it in a stable place and cool temperature. Brining will start the salt curing, but you can use additional brine solution that should be changed on a regular basis. Salt-cured require you to soak meat in water for a long time to remove the excess salt and bring it to an edible level.

Fermentation

Fermenting is fairly similar to canning, although you don't have to seal up the food and allow the entry of good bacteria. You can use acidic brine because brine helps you to control the fermentation of your food by selecting anaerobic bacteria, kill potentially harmful molds and bacteria strains to conserve your produce against breakdown.

Chapter 4: Homestead Projects

In this chapter, we are going to discuss the various projects we need to suitable Homestead.

Chicken Coop:

If you don't already have one, constructing a chicken coop will be one of your next homestead-related ventures. You can quickly create one of the scraps to give potential pet chickens a comfortable place to live. And, of course, you'll get fresh eggs every day, until you've got an avian colony on hand. That's one less item you need to buy from the store, making your home much more independent.

Construct a tool Shed:

> - **HOMESTEAD PROJECT**
>   *7 projects you need to embark on when starting your Homesteading.*
> - **DIY (DO-IT-YOUSELF) BACKYARD INITIATIVES.**
>
>   *10 projects initiative you can do by yourself.*

Constructing a small building for the keeping of your tools is essential in backyard homesteading.

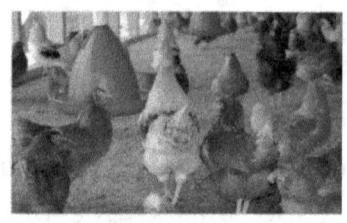

Build a Greenhouse:

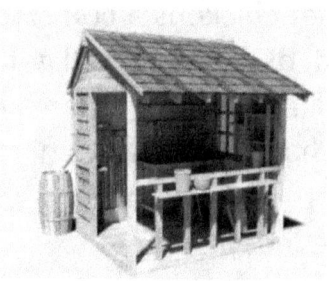

Some homesteaders get the elegance of a year-round tropical climate. If you are struggling with cold weather in the woods in your country, you might like to spend a few days constructing a greenhouse in anticipation of the chill from around edge.

Some people would have done so for as little as $50, and their indoor gardens have assisted plants to stay warm and flourish all winter long. And who wouldn't want an entire year of fresh produce?

Plant Greens
Spend a weekend bring some greenery to your farm side. For improving the appearance, you can pop up towering thrillers or massive-growing fillers into your yard. Plus, as raised by carbon dioxide-ingesting plants, more the foliage you have, the more that your Homestead contributes significantly to air purification.

Establish a Smokehouse
Homesteaders need to consider trying to maintain their food, as many items are not accessible throughout the year. You can remedy and store meats with a backyard smokehouse, and they survive longer without sacrificing any of their taste. Smoking your proteins can infuse the others even more tasty — construct this

smoker based on a cinderblock to get you to begin.

Sit by the Fire Pit:

You haven't fabricated it yet, but a DIY(Do-It-Yourself) firepit will render your Homestead even cozier. After all, not even all the land has to go to agricultural production — at least one corner of the area can be appreciated without homesteading. So, spend several days making a fire pit. Just before you 're done, assemble around and relish in the hours spent with your family members.

Make your Homestead a better place:

A few short hours of work on your farm could go a big step, So, the upcoming weekend, grab your gloves, supplies, and toolkit — it's time to create your backyard farming much successfully.

DIY HOMESTEADING BACKYARD INITIATIVES

The Homestead project development backyard:

Homesteaders, landscapers, small-scale farmers, and adventure seekers will love this compilation of 10 DIY backyard initiatives we've collected today.

You 're likely to find which you'll want to make this weekend from the chicken coop and greenhouse to a back garden that will carry all of your essential garden tools.

And no concerns about losing your savings, because all these ventures use only simple tools and materials that are easy to find.

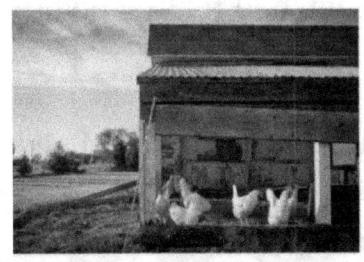

1. Coop Chicken:

Pit Explosion

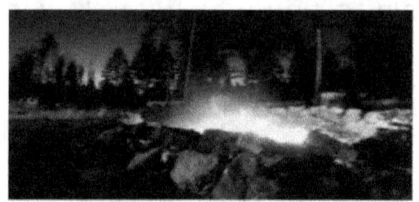

By layering tree rings and trying to fill stones or pebbles between each one, construct a warm and cozy fire pit. If at all possible, matched for any point in time of the year.

Compost bin Pallet:

Use a couple of pallets to build a super-looking dual bin system.

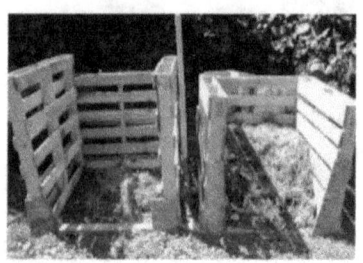

Rack of firewood:
Make an open-air firewood rack to load your firewood, and period it.

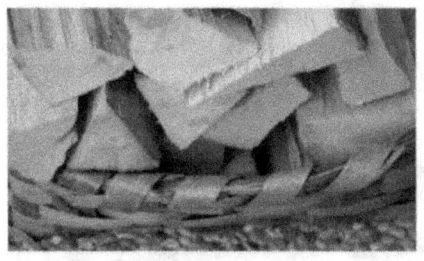

5. Scratch or Tools shed:
Create the shed for storing your tools, equipment, containers, soil planting, seeds, and much more.

6. PVC Chicken Pen:
Good initiative to maintain your chickens satisfied and reasonably comfortable from predators at the backyard.

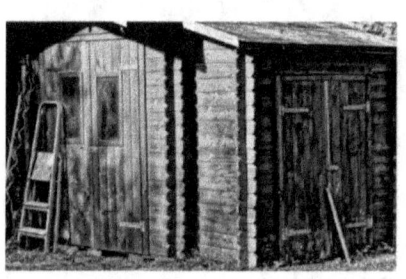

Hutch Rabbit From Wooden Pallets:

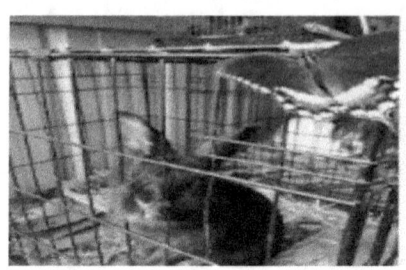

This rabbit hutch consists of 4 pallets, a rabbit floor wire roll, wooden wrenches, scrap plywood, a tow strap, hinges, as well as a latch.

Greenhouse:

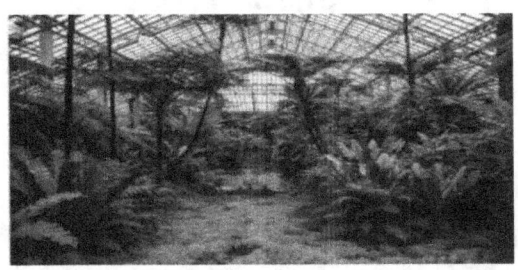

Introducing a greenhouse to your home is a great place to expand food and diverse plants throughout the year.

Smoke Shop;
If you'd like to smoke your meat, then why not create a smokehouse for yourself?

Chapter 5: Testing and Preparation of Soil Types

There are four types of soil.
Grainy
Sandy
Clay
It is ideal soil for gardening because it is well drained.
However, scientists classify soil based on its properties:
Color
The soil's color can provide information about the unprocessed material, fertility, drainage, and biotic activities. Use a garden shovel to measure the soil's color. This must be done before the sun can dry your soil, which could change the true color.
Compaction
A soil must be able breathe to be considered beneficial. This means that water can flow through it quickly and

without any difficulty. Because compressed soils don't allow much air to reach the root zone, water (e.g. rain or irrigation) tends to run-off. This increases erosion and washes away vegetation and topsoil.

Normal, loosely compressed soil allows for water to be absorbed and retained. It also releases it slowly to allow the roots of the plants to breathe. These soils are more productive as they allow plants to grow easily. These soils are dense and compacted, which can lead to less plant development, leading to more overflow.

A great indicator of soil condition is the percentage of water infiltration. The soil's most important element is sand. It feels coarse when you rub it between your thumbs and pointer fingers. It has sharp edges. Sand is not able to hold much water or nutrients.

Silt is a soil component whose size is somewhere between sand or clay. Silt is fine and chalky. The texture of silt is not sticky but smooth when it's wet. Clay is the smallest soil element. Clay can be dry and sticky, or plastic when it is soaked in water.

Clay can store many nutrients and some clay types can hold a little liquid. However, the clay's composition does not allow water and air to flow through it easily. The clay soil holds most of the liquid, and plants can't get rid of it.

Moisture content

The soil's moisture content varies depending on the type of soil, the organic material and the climate.

Although it is possible to estimate soil humidity by simply looking at the soil, this method can sometimes be a bit inaccurate. A soils laboratory is required to determine the soil moisture. A soil laboratory will dry a sample of soil on a hot plate to compare its heaviness before drying and the results after drying.

The percentage of moisture in the soil is determined based on its weight.

Organic content

The soil's organic material has a significant impact on the soil inhabitants, including animals and plants. The soil population receives the necessary nutrients from decomposing natural material. The soil is deficient in certain nutrients, and the number of soil inhabitants drops if organic materials are not added from time to time. Inflammation can determine the amount of natural material. The organic matter is made up of carbon compounds. These carbon compounds are heated to high temperatures and then converted to carbon dioxide and liquid. A dry, hard sample of material is heated up to high temperatures during the ignition process. The soil's organic matter is released as gas. This results in a change of weight that allows for the calculation of the natural substance of the sample being tested.

pH

Most people believe that rainwater has a pH of 7. It is therefore quite surprising that unpolluted rainwater is pH 6 to 6.5. This is slightly acidic. This is due to liquefied carbon dioxide, which is found in the air. It reacts with water to form a dilute acid.

It's no surprise that plants thrive in soil with the same pH. It is not surprising that many plants thrive in soil with a pH of 5.0.

Other plants such as beech, mock orange, mock orange, and asparagus can survive in soils pH 8.0. The earth becomes too limy for most plants if it has a pH higher than pH 8.5. However, soils with pH below 3.5 will not be suitable. It is important to remember that soils may differ in pH. This means that soil pH can vary within the soil but the variation is not too large.

Profil du sol

The best way to learn about soil is to get a cross-section. A soil core tool is used to do this. It's a tube that measures between 2 and 4 feet in length. The cross-section can be used to push it in.

After the tool is injected into the soil it should be turned to loosen the soil before being taken out. To identify the various layers of soil in the soil core, you can easily examine it. The sum is called a soil profile.

You can simply mark the areas where the soil's color or overall appearance changes to determine a soil horizon.

The three most important horizons in soils are the parent material, top soil, and subsoil. The top zone could contain remnants of dead and active plants, depending on where the sample was taken. The soil at the top is usually darker in color and contains more roots, organic matter and nutrients than the soil below.

The first inch of top soil might be darker in color because some nutrients have been removed by water. Natural material may not have been fully oxidized by heat or sunlight. The soil below the first inch is usually darker and contains more nutrients.

Subsoil is the next layer. It is usually a foot or so below the exterior face. The subsoil is distinguished by a lighter shade and larger roots. The subsurface layer typically contains less clay than the topsoil. The parent substance is the third and most visible level. This is composed of loose, lightly worn rocky materials from which soil is formed. It is distinguished by its limited biological activity and very few roots.

Soil Structure

This shows how the soil influences the flow of water, air and root diffusion into it. These are the descriptions of soil structure:

Blocks - These are large chunks of soil with the same number of cracks that go vertically and horizontally.

Columns - Most soil chunks and associated cracks are longer in the vertical direction than they are in the horizontal.

Granular - Granular soil is small and has the same number of cracks that go both vertically and horizontally.

Plate-like - Most soil chunks and associated cracks are longer in the flat than in the upright.

Soil Temperature

Heat in the soil plays a major role in determining how fast or slow a plant develops and whether it will live. With depth, the heat content of your soil can change dramatically.

Texture of the soil

Loam soil absorbs between a quarter of an inch and 2 inches of water per hour.

Loam is elastic, absorbent, and holds water well. Clay soil, on the other hand, is dense and compacted with very few air pockets between particles. Only a small amount of water can be accessed by plants.

Three factors out of the nine are more important than others. These are organic matter, pH and texture.

Chapter 6: Organic Production

Growing vegetables organically will require an additional set of skills and knowledge as well as certification from one of the organic authorities. They will require that to be certified as organic a set of requirements will need to be met. Organic produce may attract a price premium, however the costs are also usually greater with a higher demand for labour. To go from conventional farming to certified organic may take a few years. More information can be obtained from the individual organizations.

The Vegetable Research and Development Levy

There is a compulsory National General Vegetable Levy that must be paid at first point of sale. This levy is 0.05% of the sale price or 50c for every $100. The levy is used to fund research and development in the vegetable industry. This levy does not apply to tomatoes, potatoes, onions or mushrooms as they all have their own separate compulsory levy. Asparagus, Garlic and Melons do not pay the compulsory levy but do have voluntary levies raised to manage specific issues. If you are selling direct to the consumer it is up to you to collect and pay the levy. It will be taken out of the sale price if you sell the product on to someone else e.g. supermarket or wholesaler.

Irrigation

Water Supply And Delivery

The availability of water for irrigation is essential for vegetable production and its supply and quality will determine the area and crops that can be grown. Supply must be reliable and typical water sources include rivers or streams, channels, ground water, and farm dams. For vegetable crops generally around 6 megalitres/ha is required from planting to harvest.

Water delivery methods vary depending on where the farm is situated. Farms in controlled irrigation areas will have to pay water delivery and system maintenance fees. Water is delivered by channel or pipe. The water may not be available all year as channels may be filled only during the irrigation season of the main crops grown in the area. Water may need to be ordered or restricted to certain volume limits depending on capacity. Bores and direct pumping from rivers will also be subject to rules but there is usually more flexibility about water availability. However be aware that some streams have environmental flow requirements and once these thresholds are reached irrigation may banned until the flows increase.

An increasingly important source of water in some production areas is the use of recycled water. This is different to grey water because it has been treated to bring it back up to potable standards so it is safe to use for vegetable production. Different classes of water have different rules attached as to what they can be used for. Recycled water may have higher levels of salts and this will require careful management depending on the crop.

Water quality should be tested no matter what the source if you are considering buying a property to grow vegetables and you are unsure of the quality of the water available. Tolerance of crops to salt levels varies considerably for example beans are much less salt tolerant than broccoli.

Water Application

Application methods include drip irrigation, overhead fixed and moveable sprinklers, travelling irrigators like centre pivots and flood irrigation. Drip irrigation is the most water efficient application method but all systems have their pros and cons. Some production situations, crops or soil types may not be suited to specific irrigation methods. It is most important no matter what the method used, that an even distribution pattern of water is applied to ensure even and controlled crop growth. The method used will depend on the crop to be grown, how much water is available and the capital that can be invested. An irrigation designer is the best person to help determine what options you have.

Scheduling water application to crop needs is critical to managing irrigation. Over or under irrigation of crops can lead to quality problems, poor yields and crop loss. Monitoring the soil moisture levels is the best way to determine how much water a crop needs.

There are a number of methods that can be used to schedule irrigation, from the simple tensiometers (these require frequent monitoring and maintenance), to more expensive logging equipment such as environscan, aquaflex and neutron probes. Again check with your irrigation specialist for alternative methods. Another option is to use evapotranspiration figures. This is an estimate of evaporation and water use by crops and will indicate the amount of water used over a period of time. Evapotranspiration figures are available from some local weather stations and may be published in local newspapers or available electronically.

Monitoring of the irrigation system is important so that leaks and blockages can be picked up. The uniformity of the water application should also be checked every few seasons to detect worn nozzles. Irrigation management courses will teach you all the basics of irrigation application and system maintenance. There are run periodically by various training providers.

Climate

Climate and climatic variability is a critical factor in vegetable production and is largely beyond your control, unless you plan to establish protected cropping such as glasshouse or shade-house production. Climate will determine what crops can be grown and at what time of the year. Some crops will be frost sensitive; others will have a heat requirement or a minimum soil temperature for germination of seed.

Varieties of specific vegetable crops such as cauliflowers or lettuce are produced for particular seasonal conditions and times.

For some vegetable varieties this timing can be very specific and if they are grown outside those conditions due to poor timing or unseasonal weather, the crop may fail due to prematurely running to seed or poor head formation.

Weather

It is also important to remember that weather conditions are variable and that there are also extreme events which can affect the growing conditions and crop quality.

Weather will also have an impact on disease and insect levels. Leaf wetness increases the likelihood of some fungal diseases and this is not only due to irrigation and rain but also humidity and dew. Other conditions which can influence pest and disease incidence include temperature and wind.

Some of the adverse conditions that can cause problems include damage caused by wind or wind blown sand, as well as frost, sunburn and hail. Whilst you can't stop adverse weather there are things that can help reduce its impact, such as choosing where to plant vulnerable crops e.g. Avoiding frost hollows in frost prone months, planting wind breaks and using irrigation to reduce heat, wind or frost damage.

Some crops are more susceptible to wind, such as beans, or the spear development of asparagus can be affected. Consider the use of windbreaks and the type of windbreak for such crops.

Climate Change

It is also increasingly important to take into account the impact of potential climate change. For vegetable production the major impact is in relation to increased climate variability which may mean that there is an increased risk of crops running to seed or failing to set normal heads due to unseasonal conditions or being damaged by severe weather events. This increase in seasonal variability should be taken into account when planning planting schedules and choosing varieties. If you are establishing a new property you may want to consider the long term outlook for the area. It is likely that most parts of Victoria will become hotter and drier in the future.

Labour

The labour requirement varies significantly for different crops depending on picking frequency, pruning and training requirements. Some crops will need to be picked every couple of days or daily, others will have pruning or training requirements that may be very labour intensive. Other crops may need a once only harvest and relatively little maintenance throughout the growing period of the crop.

In choosing what crop to grow the level and frequency of labour needed to manage the crop should be taken into account. For labour intensive crops, production on a larger scale will require significantly more labour and so may not give the economies of scale that might have been expected.

Harvesting

Harvest labour can be a significant consideration when deciding to grow vegetables. You may need a consistent supply of labour or many hands all at once or something in between.

The crop you choose will dictate the type of labour you need. Crops generally fall into one of four categories

• Harvested by machinery: These do not have a high demand for labour but the capital outlay for the machinery may be significant. Examples are potatoes, corn, carrots and processing tomatoes.

• Harvested by hand once: Labour demands for these crops are generally lower. Depending on the size of the operation these may be managed by a family unit. Considerations will depend on the perishability of the crop and how quickly it needs to be harvested after it matures. An example of this are pumpkins.

• Harvested by hand with multiple picks and/or multiple cropping: Labour demand for these crops will vary depending on the size of the area planted and the number of picks required. Broccoli for example will usually have 2-3 picks and crops are also planted sequentially every one or two weeks to provide continuity of supply throughout the season.

• Harvested by hand continuously: Crops may need pruning or training as well as harvesting. These crops may produce over a whole season or for extended periods with sequential plantings. Examples of these crops include fresh tomatoes, squash, eggplant, asparagus and snow peas.

Regular work makes it easier to keep good employees but can cause problems if there is limited labour.

Needing labour all at once or semi regularly can mean spending more time on training of new staff each time you need workers.

Cooling and Other Handling Requirements

Some of the things to consider after harvest include does your crop require refrigeration, ice, or post-harvest treatments such as washing, trimming or fungicides. Just placing product in the cool room is usually not enough to get the harvested crop down to a suitable temperature before transport. The outer product may be cool but product in the middle of the box or pallet may have only been reduced a couple of degrees. Additional cooling infrastructure may be needed such as forced air cooling or hydro-cooling. The whole post harvest cooling chain is only as strong as the weakest link and poor post harvest handling will result in a rapid loss in quality and significant product loss.

Crops will need to be packed and graded according to size and/or colour depending on the type of crop. This means that there may be a requirement for packing and grading lines. These issues will also affect the amount of labour needed.

Some products before being sent to market will need to be washed for phytosanitary requirements or for appearance, for example, to remove soil on potatoes. Water quality is also a factor and there may need to be treatment of the water, e.g. filtering or chlorination for it to be suitable as wash water.

The crop will need to be stored prior to sale or shipment and most vegetable crops will require storage in a coolroom. Even crops that do not need cold storage may need some treatment, for example onions and pumpkins need to be cured if they are to store well.

What You Need to Know

If you are considering converting to vegetable production from other forms of horticulture there are a few things to be aware of.

• Full time vegetable farms generally involve more consistent labour throughout the year than tree or vine crops because there is no winter dormancy.

• Irrigation systems for trees and vines will not necessarily be suitable for vegetable production e.g. Emitter spacings may be too far apart.

• Crop prices are more volatile than perennial crops because there can be huge variation in the amount of a particular crop planted each year and seasonal conditions in production areas can have a big effect on supply

• There is very a strong sense of competition among vegetable farmers and peer support may be difficult to get.

• Ground that has recently grown another horticulture crop may struggle to support vegetable production before a suitable fallow period.

• Generally vegetables grown between rows of perennial crops will mean that both crops suffer particularly if on the one irrigation system as they usually have different water requirements and spray programs.

• Vegetable growers continually crop throughout a season to take into account the seasonal variation of peaks and troughs in supply. Do not expect that the production of any one crop will necessarily return a profit. That will depend upon supply and demand at harvest as well as the crop and quality you produce.

Types of Fertilizer You Should Try

Take a stroll through the plant fertilizer aisle at your local garden center and you'll be met with a dizzying array of fertilizer options.

Take a stroll through the plant fertilizer aisle at your local garden center and you'll be met with a dizzying array of fertilizer options. The different types of fertilizers aren't necessarily better than one another. They're each meant to address certain plant growth needs. Many gardeners use a combination of fertilizer types over the course of the year. Generally, an all-purpose fertilizer is just fine for basic gardening. Always follow manufacturer's instructions carefully when applying fertilizer, over fertilization burns plants.

Granular Fertilizer

Granular fertilizers are dry fertilizers that usually come in pellet form and must be either worked into or watered into the soil. These are applied with an automatic spreader or a fertilizer shaker container. Granular fertilizers are best suited for fertilizing larger areas. You can buy them in slow-release, controlled-release, and quick-release formulas designed to work for different amounts of time.

Slow-Release Fertilizer

Slow- or gradual-release fertilizers are excellent for quick-color plants. These products feature special coatings that gradually release nutrients, usually over a period of three to nine months. The fertilizer label will clearly specify the time frame. Slow-release products frequently are already blended into bagged potting mixes, both soilless and soil-base types. If you purchase mixes that don't contain fertilizer, add it prior to planting. As the name suggests, it may take some time before you see results, but slow-release fertilizers prompt steadier growth. Midway through the growing season, if needed, you can work more slow-release fertilizer into the soil.

Liquid Fertilizer (or Soluble Fertilizer)

Liquid fertilizers are available as powders or in bottled liquid solutions. Dissolved in water, soluble fertilizers deliver a quick nutrient burst. They're easy to handle and store and contain a high percentage of macronutrients per weight. In soil with organic matter, nutrients from a soluble fertilizer are retained. But in sandy soil or soilless mixes, nutrients move out of root zones quickly when more water washes through the soil. Most liquid fertilizers are poured onto soil. Some are sprayed onto leaves, which absorb nutrients.

Organic Fertilizer

Organic fertilizers include compost and manure, which provide slow-release nitrogen. These fertilizers typically are used with planting beds or large containers like half-barrel planters. They improve soil structure, encourage soil microbes and earthworms, and contain a high level of micronutrients that plants need to grow. Some organic fertilizers, such as bonemeal, blood meal, or cottonseed meal, are concentrated. A small amount of these materials offers a large nutrient boost, which explains their often higher price. Although meal fertilizers are a good organic choice, they require microbes to break them down. That means they can't provide readily available nutrients during cold seasons when microbes are inactive. This is why it's important to prepare your plants ahead of time, in the fall.

How to Use Fertilizer and Water Together

You can apply liquid fertilizer to plants directly with your garden hose by adding a hose end sprayer attachment. The water flowing through the hose dilutes the concentrate. These are available as fixed rate sprayers, which release a set amount of fertilizer per gallon of water each time, or adjustable sprayers, which have a dial that lets you control the settings.

Common Fertilizer Issues

Most plants give clues when available nutrients are insufficient to fuel growth.Watch foliage carefully. When nitrogen is scarce, leaves turn yellow. Too little phosphorus causes leaves to turn reddish or purple. Older leaves burn and drop when potassium is in short supply. Other symptoms of nutrient deficiency include weak or slow growth and smaller leaves and flowers. Note that temperature shifts, insufficient light, and overwatering can also cause some of these symptoms. Troubleshoot light and watering habits first so you don't accidentally over-fertilize your plants.

Tips and Tricks

• Fence your garden. A fence, besides keeping out rabbits and other hungry animals, helps define your garden visually. Poultry netting is inexpensive and effective. To keep animals from burrowing under your fence, bend the bottom foot of fencing to the outside of the garden to lay right on top of the ground. Unless deer are a threat in which case you need a fence 5 or more feet high a 2- or 3-foot-high fence should be adequate.

• Make your garden pretty. Yes, it's a vegetable garden, but even vegetable gardens can be pretty. Wooden pickets can obscure and dress up a poultry netting fence. An arbor, with climbing beans or grapes, can dress up your garden gate. Soften the fence line with an outside border planting of shrubs, perhaps something decorative and edible such as red currants or blueberries. Beauty will also draw you into your garden.

• Planning your garden in four dimensions is a way to harvest more from limited space. Rather than single, widely spaced rows, plant in wide (3 to 4 feet) beds (a second dimension). Rather than keeping everything at ground level, let your vegetables those that can grow up (a third dimension). Pole beans and tomatoes can be trained up bamboo or metal poles, and peas and cucumbers can be trained up fences even that fence that encloses your garden. For the fourth dimension time use transplants for tomatoes, peppers, eggplants, and cucumbers, and plant shorter-season vegetables to follow those that finish early or start late, such as lettuce following early bush beans.

- Pay attention to fertilizing and watering. Spread a balanced organic fertilizer over the ground in late winter at the rate suggested on the container. Or, if existing vegetation is growing well, use soybean meal at 2 pounds per 100 square feet. Or apply an inch depth of compost. Set out a straight-sided can to measure water, and turn on the sprinkler once a week so the combination of rain and sprinkling equal an inch depth of water in that can.
- Weed regularly and frequently. Weeds are much easier to kill and haven't had time to spread many seeds when they are small.
- Grow vegetables that you like to eat, and choose the best-tasting varieties.
- For future successes, thoroughly clean up old plants when they're finished or at the end of the season, and move plants around the garden so they don't grow in the same spot for a couple of years.

Chapter 7: Let's Start! The Basic Steps To Growing In Containers

Now that you are apprised of the important considerations that a gardener who plans to venture into a container gardening may face, we may now look into the fundamental part of the project-the engagement into container gardening itself.

You are now in the phase of initializing your vision of having home-grown food even if you are a city-dweller. Here are the key tasks to kick start your own container garden.

Choose what you're going to grow.

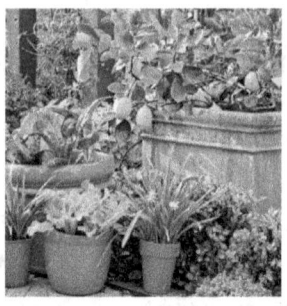

The first thing that you must keep in mind is the kind of plants that you want to grow in your garden and the seasons of your location. You have a lot of choices to pick from but limit this according to your needs and the complexity of taking care of the plants. Since it's a container garden that you would like to maintain, herbs like basil, rosemary, sage and mint are practical. Veggies like red and green lettuce and even tomatoes will also thrive in containers. A more detailed elaboration of what you can grow in pots can be found in the next chapters.

Location...location...Choosing the Best Spot

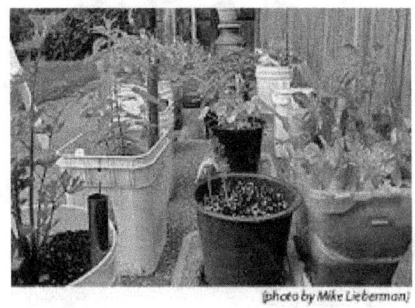
(photo by Mike Lieberman)

Plants need sunshine in order to live. It is a common guide; flowering plants, water plants, and fruiting vegetables necessitate at least eight hours of sunshine per day to thrive well. If its root vegetables, they can do with six hours, and for leafy vegetables including herbs, they should at least receive four hours of sun. As some plants may require more shade, do a little research on a specific plant you want to grow because not all vegetation requires the same degree of sunlight.

Prepare Your Gardening Gear

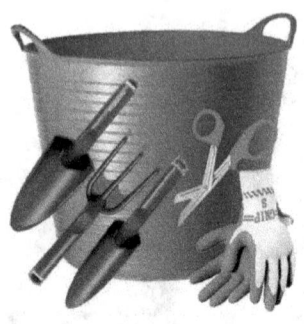

Gathering your gear is not too difficult when you want to start container gardening. It requires a small number of tools. It is just standard to have gloves, a trowel and a hand fork or claw. In case of plants that may require pruning, a simple pair of kitchen scissors or shears may come in handy. Just remember to keep your tools at their clean state and their blades in a good level of sharpness to make them easier to use.

Find Containers that You can Effectively Utilize

In choosing a container or pots, you can make use of just about any container including terra cotta (commonly known as clay pots), plastic pots or containers, wooden barrels, cable baskets lined with moss or coconut husks, ceramic pots of various colors and sizes, planter boxes, and even cement blocks. If you plan to recycle old materials worthy to be transformed into containers, do not use those that have held toxic chemicals if you plan to grow edible plants in them.

Since any container can be of use for a small-scale garden, just make sure that they can effectively hold water and they facilitate drainage. If a material to be used a s container has no drain, drill multiple holes at the bottom to allow water to flow. This idea to some extent made people consider using even the strangest of containers like old boots, old tires turned inside out and even used toilet bowls, among others. Well, as long as plant growth will be facilitated, any material will do as a container. Just remember that, containers made from permeable materials like clay or wood, lose dampness too quickly, but let air movement into the roots effectively. Metal, plastic, and glazed containers are non-porous—but they hold water much longer, however they restrict air movement. So making drainage holes is important.

The weight and size of your pots is also a consideration particularly if they will have a tendency to be mover around to facilitate easier lifting. Bigger and taller plants may need larger containers, and to move them easier you may add wheelies for easier mobility. Use a slightly larger pot to reduce times of maintenance and let the soil hold more moisture. With a larger pot, the roots of large plants will not be crowded and will be easily accommodated. If you plan to plant vegetables peppers, eggplants, tomatoes, beans or cabbages make sure to use bigger pots.

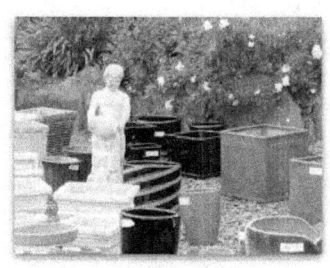

Many vegetables, herbs, and flowers will not be prolific if they are allowed to wither. Containers that are small in size carry less moisture especially when the roots are congested. They will need more care during summer. Consider using a bigger container that can carry more soil to hold moisture and reduce maintenance.

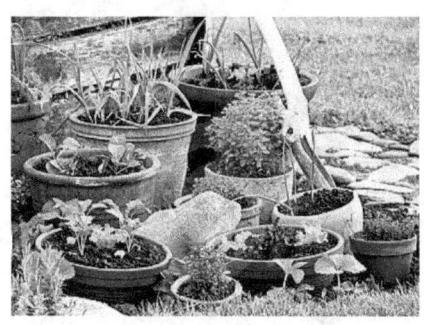

The size of the container must be able to hold the roots of the plants when fully matured. Vegetables like tomatoes, eggplant, pepper, cucumbers, cabbage, and beans will need a container that can hold at least 5 gallons of soil. Three-gallon containers will be enough for beets, carrots, green onions and lettuce. For most herbs and radish plants, one gallon or lesser containers will suffice. For flowering plants, the larger the mass of the roots, a larger container will be required.

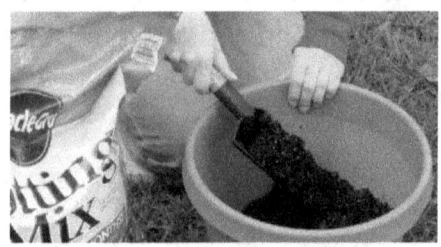

The Best Type of Soil You Can use
Another significant thing you will need to start your container garden is the soil. Soil is very important to plants and their type

and availability depends from region to region. The type of soil best for plants directly related to the plant you wish to grow. Sand, silt and clay are the three common types of earth, Sandy loam soil is the perfect mixture for plants. Sometimes you need to use compost or add peat moss to improve the quality of the soil.

In the cities, good soil may not be easily available. If you need to soil for your garden, your destination is a nursery or store for agricultural supply. Potting soil is highly preferred than the native earth that you can get from the ground because the former has more water-retentive capabilities and is sure to be free from weeds and disease. The mix may also have a balanced mixture of nutrients ideal for the plants and are well-suited to adapt to most types of plants that you want to place in containers.

Make use of good soil mixes by choosing that are free of organisms, weeds and disease. Make sure to never reuse old potting soil previously used in an earlier season because it may pass existing disease and organisms to your next plants. Soil with a slightly acidic pH as well as porous enough to hold water and nutrients is ideal for plants.

Nurseries and specialty stores will offer potting soil that contain pasteurized soil, vermiculite, perlite, sphagnum peat moss and composted manure. These ingredients are ideal and will improve the quality of your plants.

You can also opt to use soilless mixes since they contain a lot of the same components as potting soil. However soil less mix is much lighter because they are devoid of heavy soil. In it are peat moss and/or ground bark which hold nutrients and water; vermiculite meant for water retention; and perlite that allows for air movement. The light-weight features may be a problem for top-heavy vegetation so to resolve this place coarse sand up to ten percent of the pot's volume.

Just take note that plants intended for the indoors need a different kind of soil. To simply scoop some soil from a source like your yard may not be a good idea due to the bacteria that may do more harm than good to your houseplants. You can use commercial potting soil or do any of the two options:

One is to sterilize the soil. By placing your outdoor soil in a baking sheet, heat it in the oven at 180 degrees. This will take care of the bacteria, weeds and other organisms. To make the soil plant worthy, after pasteurization, add peat moss or sand. Or, instead of buying from a store, you can make your own soilless mix. Here is a good mixture recipe which will create a light-weight potting plant mix. Put together equal amounts of peat moss, sand and perlite (and/or vermiculite). Instead of sand you can use bark or coconut husk or coir instead of peat moss. It depends on your personal preference. For the nutrients, add small amounts of fertilizer and ground limestone. Mix the ingredients thoroughly and store in an air-lock container.

Chapter 8: Plant Nutrition & Troubleshooting

How to Prevent Nutrient Lockout

Hydroponics growers face many challenges, but nutrient lockout is the most difficult. It can cause crop death and lower yields.

What does Nutrient Lockout mean?

When crops are not able to absorb the nutrients that should be available in hydroponics systems, it is called "nutrient lockout" or "nutrient lock". It can be difficult to identify the problem for first-time growers. If it isn't resolved quickly, it could lead to the death of many crops.

When nutrient lock is occurring, plants can look healthy and green until they develop major symptoms on their leaves and roots. Many plants will then begin to wilt and eventually die.

Is Nutrient Lock caused by a System's Nutrient Level?

A high level of nutrients in hydroponics solutions can cause nutrient lockout. This is ironic. This is what it looks like. Oversaturation can cause a chain reaction which ultimately reduces the ability of plants to absorb nutrients.

The result is that the plants become starved, despite the fact that there are plenty of nutrients in the water. The grower must take immediate steps to release the nutrients and save his crops if there is a lockout. Crop death is possible if this happens.

Is Nutrient lockout caused by an improper pH balance?

This is because fertilizers are not always applied correctly. This is because your plants may appear underfed, even if you add fertilizer regularly to your system.

It can sometimes be difficult to get the pH balance right because it is often dependent on the plant. Certain plants are more sensitive to a particular nutrient than others. This can lead to a deficiency in absorption of other nutrients.

Manganese absorption is a good example. Manganese is more easily absorbed by plants roots when it reaches pH 5. Calcium and magnesium should be left out at the same pH level. You, the grower need to determine the pH level that is most beneficial for your plants.

You can do this by carefully observing the pH trend of your hydroponics system, and then matching the nutrients solution to the appearance of the plants. You can make small adjustments to the amount of fertilizer that you add to your system each day to have a significant impact on the overall system.

What does Nutrient Lockout look like?

Because nutrient lockout refers to nutritional deficiency and poor nutrient utilization, it is important that you look out for these symptoms. The following are the most frequent signs of nutrient deficiencies:

1. Stunted growth. Stunted growth is characterized by a smaller overall structure, smaller flowers, fruits and

leaves, rather than dense. Compare the appearances of mature plants to determine if you are on the right path.

2. Leaves. Deficiency of different minerals such as magnesium can often be seen in yellowing leaves. A yellowing of plant matter could also indicate too many salts or pH imbalances.

a. Pink and yellow speckling may be seen on some plants. The leaves would have a border of green but would show obvious yellow and pink spots, particularly in the middle.

Other signs of nutrient deficiencies in plants' leaves include:

- Browning and drying of the leaves' edges.
- Curling and browning.

Foliage is a combination of a dull and some yellowing.

The leaves might not appear as jaunty or erect as they should. Some leaves may appear paler and dry.

Reddish-brown tones may be seen in some cases along with a dull pallor and some yellowing.

How to Fix Nutrient Lockout

Before you do anything to fix a potential nutrient leakage, ensure that you compare the appearance of your plants with the results of any nutrient solutions you've used. Before you can diagnose the problem, there must be strong correlation. You could inadvertently do more damage to your plants.

After a few days of testing you can determine if there is a nutrient blockage. If so, flush the system. Flushing helps remove excess salts and stabilizes the pH. It also gives your crops a chance for 'breathing' and reactivates their nutrient uptake.

This is common with hydroponics systems as salts build up in the water while we add more fertilizer. The lockout occurs when there is no choice but to add nutrients.

Pure water can be used to flush your system. It might also be worthwhile to conduct a thorough inspection of your entire system during this time.

Make sure to inspect the pumps, pipes, and drains. Blockages, fungal growth, and other issues can cause long-term problems. This is why you should take this "break time" to ensure that your hydroponics system works as it should.

Prevention

We don't enjoy having to treat our crops often. This is a serious problem and one incident with nutrient lockout can ruin a whole season. This problem can be prevented.

1. Use buffering solutions to adjust the pH level. A buffering formula is often included in high quality liquid fertilizers. This helps to keep the pH level of your water stable.

2. Flushing solutions should be used to reduce stress on plants and the entire system. Flushing solutions are designed to remove excess salts from the system, as they (re)circulate. You can still flush the system with water, but you'll get better results if there are active compounds present.

3. Use RO (reverse-osmosis water) whenever possible. The chemical balance of your hydroponics system may be affected by purified water, which has a lower level of common chemical compounds.

4. You should monitor your pH and EC levels daily and keep track of the data. This will enable you to see trends over weeks or months and allow you calculate the average using this data.

What does Flushing mean in Hydroponics?

Flushing refers to the process of cleaning out hydroponics systems in order to protect the health of the crops being grown there. Flushing is possible before harvest but should only be done if the crops are in distress.

Why flush?

Flushing is one way to relieve plant stress, as was already mentioned. Flushing is a physical process that removes salts from the water.

Salt buildup in hydroponics systems is natural because the liquid fertilizers are actually separated once they have been applied to water.

Some nutrients are lost due to the action of water, plants, and eventually the nutrient content gets higher and higher. The dreaded "nutrient lock" is what happens when too many nutrients are in the water.

How to flush

You can flush your hydroponics system in many ways, but this is the easiest.

You can add steps if necessary, but this process is sufficient.

Removing old water and draining it

First, drain the main tank of your hydroponics system. You can pour water into a traditional garden if it is still full of nutrients.

Drain the reservoir until the bottom is dry. You can use smaller systems that require buckets or other small containers. The main tub from which the nutrients are circulated must also be empty.

Remove and scrape algae

It's time for you to clean the tub or reservoir. It is best to flush it with water continuously, turning off the pump and allowing the drain to open. This will ensure that no visible components are left on the bottom or walls.

Although salts are not colorless, they can cause havoc in your system if they combine with your water. Hydroponics systems that have been in use for a while may show signs of algae.

Use a scraper to remove visible fungi or algae. You can manually remove as much gunk as you can and flush the rest. After you have scrubbed or scraped, rinse it all. It is important to remove all visible parts from the system.

Flushing agent

After the system has been thoroughly cleaned and flushed, you can close the drain and refill your system with water. Turn on the pump to start circulating the water.

This one can be done with plain water, but it is better to use purified water or filtered water if you are unable to. For hydroponics system cleaning, purified water is better. Here is where you can add the appropriate amount of flushing agents to your system.

Flushing agents are used to kill bacteria, fungi and algae, as well as help remove other impurities from the water.

There is no one way to apply a flushing agent. Follow the manufacturer's instructions for the best results. You can also match flushing agent to the system you have and the water available.

Drain the system once more with the flushing agent. Next, inspect all parts to determine if any sediment, molds, or algae remain. If necessary, perform another rinse and then move on to the next step.

Stabilization of the hydroponics system

This is the longest part of the flushing process. You should again fill the set with water. Make sure you have enough water to reach the optimal level in each tub or vat.

You can add or remove a flushing agent. If in doubt, refer to the manufacturer's instructions again. Adjust the pH and EC as necessary. To be ready, the system must have the correct level of EC/PHP. All pumps should be turned on and everything should run for 24 hours.

Drain the whole setup and then refill with purified water after 24 hours. You can then operate the setup the same way you would normally.

Unless you notice problems with your pH or EC levels or if your plants show signs of nutrient locking out, there will not be a need for another flush. If you do, then repeat the entire process to remove any salts.

Other tips to improve flushes

1. To ensure everything is in perfect condition, a flush should be performed within a week of harvesting. These should be checked and measured daily to ensure that you are aware of any fluctuations. Hydroponics monitoring software is also recommended to observe trends over

time so that you can predict whether something is going down or not.

2. Flushing your harvest before harvesting will have an added benefit: It will enhance the flavor of your harvest. The water's nutrient level can affect the taste of your crops. Purified, balanced water will improve the flavor of any crops you plan to harvest. Hydroponic crops with bitter aftertastes often indicate an excess of one or two nutrients. This will then be evident in the plants once they are eaten.

3. If you notice brown or curled leaves, a flush might be the best thing to do. This is often a sign of nutrient lock. It can cause severe damage to any crop.

4. It is generally better to flush with purified water rather than tap water. Tap water contains minerals and chemicals that are used to remove bacteria and metals from the water. These chemicals can cause problems with your hydroponics system, and may even cause it to fail. You can use large system filters to filter out impurities in tap water before using it in

your hydroponics system. It is easier to balance the pH and EC levels of water that is purer. This will make your job much easier in the long-term.

5. You should be careful when using organic grow media such as coconut coir. They may become malnourished during flushing. We won't flush your plants and keep their roots dry during this process. For most media, the flushing period should be less than seven days.

6. The resin glands of your plants can be inspected for signs of ripeness. When the plants are ready to be harvested, resin glands will begin to change in color.

Use Fulvic or Humic as a Plant Fertilizer

The "missing link" in agricultural production is humic and fulvic acid. Agriculturists, as well as experts, are only now beginning to see the benefits of their application in both hydroponics and conventional farming. These two acids are crucial for maintaining healthy systems.

Both fulvic and humic acids are part of the same chemical family, which benefits crops equally. Humic acid can be water-soluble and can take on a dark brown or black color.

Fulvic acid, on the other hand is a low molecular-weight humic acid with a lighter color. It's typically yellow or light brown when reconstituted and applied in a hydroponics system.

Since they don't contain nutrients, humic and fulvic acid are not fertilizers. However, they are extremely potent soil conditioners and system conditioners that can be used by both hydroponics and conventional farmers.

HA and FA should always be used together with nutrient mixtures and/or fertilizers for hydroponics systems.

Although hydroponics systems don't have soil, FA and HA can still be used to supplement the nutrients in the system. These compounds are still very effective even without soil.

Use Fulvic and Humic as Plant Fertilizers
Promotes Beneficial Fungi

Humic acid is an agricultural revolutionizer because it promotes the growth and development of many types of beneficial fungi. This includes the well-known mycorrhizal mushrooms.

You may be aware that root diseases can develop in hydroponics systems because the roots of the plants constantly come in contact with the nutrients solution.

You can create the ideal environment for your crops without the risk of root problems and mold growth by adding humic acid, fullvic acid, and mycorrhizal mushrooms to the mix.

It increases cell growth, elongation, and nutrient uptake

Humic acid can buffer the environment that could affect plants and improve nutrient absorption by up to 40%. It can also prevent the development of the terrible condition known as nutrient lock.

One or both of these conditions can trigger nutrient lock: too many minerals salts are present in the system, or pH levels have fluctuated to the point that plant roots cannot use available nutrients.

The nutrient solution contains a lot of nutrients, but the plants are not getting enough, which can lead to plant malnutrition. Humic acid can improve plant nutrient uptake by increasing the permeability in the plant's cells.

It also contains an auxin-like promoter that increases cellular elongation. If you are looking for a bigger harvest, there is no reason to not apply humic acid or fulvic acid.

Your Nutrient Solution's Quality is Improved

Humic acid has a high CEC (cation exchange capacity). What does this mean? It binds to micro-elements in soil or water, and then holds them in a form that plants can absorb directly for nourishment and growth.

It contains many negatively charged ions, which attach to positively charged cations in its nutrient solution. These cations are rich in nutrients such as calcium, magnesium, and other minerals. In other words, humic acid basically removes nutrients from the solution so that your plants can use them.

HA and FA are a way to turbo-charge your system's ability to sustain its crops. Chelation is the process of binding negatively charged electrons to positively charged cations.

Although soil humus, peat moss and both contain natural FA/HA, the commercial version can provide up to five times that amount. It is possible to see the benefits of regular application of humic acids to crops, particularly if they have struggled for a while.

Regulates the Depletion Zone

Because plants absorb macro and micro nutrients continuously, it is possible to easily deplete the area around the roots.

HA and FA reduce the depletion zone because they can bind positively charged cations. They essentially act like large storage boxes that allow plants to reach inside and grab nutrients when they need them.

The natural affinity of humic acids to plant roots is what makes them so attractive.

This process happens repeatedly throughout the day. With enough humic acid applied, you can expect a truly abundant harvest even if your crops haven't been grown hydroponically for a while.

Hydroponic Media Improved

Experts have recently discovered that humic acid can improve the quality of grow media like clay. This is the base material for expanded clay pellets.

Clay can become softer, porous and more aerobic if it is exposed to humic acid continuously. Expanded clay pellets are often mixed with vermiculite or perlite because of its poor record in aerating the roots. Hydroponics is not a great place to be. Low oxygen levels can lead to many problems that can severely impact the quality of your harvest.

It is remarkable that, despite clay not being organic matter per se but still yields complex compounds in humic acid. Experts have discovered that clay can drain moisture faster after being exposed to humic acid for a long time.

Let's not forget, humic acid can be used to stimulate plant growth and increase nutrient uptake. They can also help remove heavy metals and toxic chemical compounds from the plants' immediate environment.

Humic acids can be applied to any type of farmer, whether you're a traditional farmer or a modern hydroponics gardener who is constantly on the lookout in the latest innovations for soil-less cultivation.

How to Apply Humic Acids

You can buy both powdered and liquid Humic Acids. It is possible to add the powder to hydroponics systems, but it is best to mix the powder with water before adding the rest of the nutrients.

If you have liquid humic acids, you can add it to your nutrient reservoir. You don't need to use large amounts of humic acids to stabilize your system, unlike nutrients and fertilizers.

A little goes a long way in humic acid. Adding more won't make your plants any healthier. To maintain the supply, make sure you reapply every so often.

For foliar spraying, you can add 20 mg/ml to 20 liters water. General system maintenance: Dissolve 100 mg/ml humic acid for every 100ml water.

What does Hydroponic Nutrients' NPK Fertilizer Ratio mean?

Understanding Plant Nutrition

Hydroponics growers need to understand how plant nutrition works. When you use a soilless system, you're not just adding fertilizer; you are giving the plants everything they need.

The soil naturally contains minerals and decaying organic material, so fertilizers are only an addition to the crop's nutrition. Hydroponics systems require only water to add nutrients.

Two types of nutrients are consumed by plants. They differ in their requirements to sustain plant life. Macronutrients are nutrients plants consume in greater quantities. Micronutrients are nutrients plants absorb in much lower amounts but are still essential for plant life.

What does NPK mean?

NPK is an acronym for three essential plant nutrients. They are nitrogen, phosphorous and potassium. These are the three most important macronutrients plants need to thrive.

It is important to get the NPK fertilizer ratio just right. Micronutrients are also very important but not the main focus.

Each fertilizer brand will have its own NPK rate, so be sure to check before you buy fertilizer. NPK stands for the percentage of potassium, phosphorous and nitrogen in that fertilizer.

There are many fertilizers that are not the same. Not all fertilizers are created equal. Hydroponics can be improved by understanding the NPK ratios. Plants that are properly nourished will have a greater harvest and will grow healthier.

It is simple to read the NPK ratio. Let's assume that fertilizers have a NPK ratio of 7-9-5. This simply means that your plants will receive seven percent nitrogen and nine percent phosphorous.

This is due to the larger mix of nutrients in fertilizers.

One fertilizer may contain more than 20 different plant nutrients. A fertilizer ratio of 9% is important because it allows you to compare the amount of each nutrient to the rest.

What is the best NPK ratio for vegetable states?

The most effective NPK ratio for plants in their vegetative stage is the 7-9-5 ratio. This ratio is commonly used in fertilizers that are called "grow", as it helps to develop dense, green, and lush foliage.

This ratio increases the plant's vegetative state. Additional nitrogen can help increase the plant's growth until harvest. Hydroponic fertilizers and nutrient solutions marked "grow" or "vegetative" can be used to accelerate the maturation of your crops.

What is the best NPK ratio for flowering/fruit stage?

The flowering stage refers to the point when crops produce their fruits and vegetables. Depending on the plants that you have, flowering/fruiting could mean different things depending on which cultivars are being taken care of.

This is when hydroponics growers prepare for harvest. Since the sixties agriculture has come a long way. Growers have now access to many fertilizers and other compounds that can help them control the various growth phases of their plants.

Plants generally require more phosphorous during the fruiting/flowering stage than they do nitrogen.

For healthy root structures and fruit and flower growth, phosphorous is essential. Potassium is the most important nutrient you should be looking for, in addition to phosphorous.

At this point, it would be beneficial to find a fertilizer with a 0-0-3 NPK ratio. This is specifically designed for large quantities of fruits in all plants. You can also use one-part formulations that are specifically designed for bloom or fruit. These have been modified to increase fruit production.

These have been modified to increase fruit production.

14. You may have noticed that the nitrogen content has dropped to five percent. However, the levels of phosphorous, potassium, and magnesium have increased to fifteen percent to fourteen percent.

Why is it that plants don't need as much nitrogen in the flowering/fruiting stage?

This is because plants in the vegetative stage are more likely to store and absorb enough nitrogen over the long-term. Your crops will not be benefited by giving them more nitrogen - but they will benefit from potassium and phosphorous.

What other NPK Ratios are used?

There are so many NPK ratios out there that it would be impossible to list them all. We can however discuss the most popular to give you an idea of what you should look for when shopping for liquid fertilizers.

General Purpose

A general purpose ratio can be used to determine the vegetative state of crops. It can also be substituted for bloom formula if it isn't available.

NPK ratios for general purpose fertilizers are 10-10-10. General purpose fertilizers should not be used if there is already a system in place and you are only adding to it with equal amounts of potassium, phosphorous and nitrogen.

Bloom Boosters:

You may have heard of bloom boosters, or hyper-chargers, that can be used in the fruiting phase of plants. You should be aware that bloom boosters can cause serious side effects in certain cultivars. The NPK ratio for bloom boosters is 0-50-30.

These mixtures contain a lot of potassium and phosphorous. If used incorrectly, they can cause pH changes in hydroponics systems and even nutrient lock. Experts warn you that misuse of bloom boosters could lead to the exact opposite effect of what you thought.

If you give your plants too much, and you are unable to balance the system, you might end up with a drastically reduced harvest with smaller fruits and stunted growings.

This can also be caused by nutrient locking, which is when the system has too many nutrients. Ironically, the plants are shut down and malnutrition is a result. This can be disastrous because you've been waiting all season for harvest.

Transition Ratios

Crops do not jump from the vegetative stage (or vertical growth stage), to the blooming/fruiting phase instantly. Many websites overlook the transition phase, which is actually the middle phase.

The transition stage is the middle stage in between the vegetative and blooming/fruiting stages. We recommend you combine your flower formula and your vegetative formula during this stage. Combine fifty percent of each batch to speed up the process of blooming/fruiting.

How do you know if the vegetative stage is finished for your plants? It's simple: check to see if your plants still grow in height. If the height growth stops, your plants will be ready to begin growing flowers or fruits.

Be excited! This is the moment we've been waiting for: Your crops are getting ready to bear fruits. Once you're certain that the vegetative stage has ended, you can shift to your preferred fruiting/blooming method to increase your yield.

DIY Fertilizer Nutrients: Making Your Own Nutrient Solution At Home

You may have thought about creating your own hydroponics system to feed your plants if you are like us. You are not the only one, there are many growers who supplement their systems using DIY nutrients.

As long as you understand the science behind fertilizers and the workings of micronutrients, there is almost always no harm. There is also an additional benefit. You can save money by sourcing your nutrients correctly. Over time, these savings could translate into upgrades to your hydroponics system. It's quite a nice idea, isn't it?

The basics of plant nutrition

Hydroponics or soil, the process of nutrient absorption is the same. The nutrients are brought into contact with the roots and the roots react with them to absorb the nutrients in forms that can then be used by plants.

Plants need two types of nutrients: micronutrients or macronutrients. While macronutrients can be consumed in greater quantities, micronutrients, which are essential for cell regulation, growth and other important functions, are needed in much smaller amounts. Collectively, plant nutrients are called "salts."

When you hear the term "salt concentration", it simply refers to the amount or concentration of nutrients in a particular environment.

Chemistry teaches us that solutions can have different levels of concentration and that concentration is affected by the volume of the solution. The concentration of a teaspoonful of nutrients in water would differ between a glass and a five-gallon jug.

Measuring salts

It is crucial to ensure that the water is clean. Contaminated water could contain chemicals or other minerals that can cause damage to plants.

This isn't vanity. Tap water contains fluorine and calcium as well as other compounds that can alter the water's chemistry. Water filtered by a reverse osmosis system will be more balanced than tap water.

It is best to use a calibrated digital scale to measure nutrients individually.

The overall balance of the system will be affected by small fluctuations in each nutrient. You don't want to accidentally cause a nutrient block because you have added too much salt.

Dissolving Salts

It is easy to dissolve salts in water. You will notice that they disappear immediately after you add them. Slowly add the salts one at a while. Only add the next salt after the previous one is completely dissolved.

To help dissolve the salts, you can swirl the water around a bit. It was fun! It's now time to test how healthy your nutritional solution is. Use a pH meter to check the pH of your nutrient solution.

The pH level that is ideal should not be higher than 7 but not lower than 5.5. Some plants are not able to tolerate pH levels above 6.5. You should monitor your plants closely to ensure they are adjusting to the mix you have made.

You can flush if the old pH adjustments are not working. However, only after you have exhausted all other options to break the nutrient locking.

This is the step-by-step process:

1. Decide how much nutrient mixture you want to mix. Is it a liter, two-liters, or a gallon of nutrient formula? You will need to decide how much you want and then find the right container size for it.
1. You should ensure that the container is clean and free of any possible contaminants.

b. Both food-grade plastic and glass containers can be used, but it is more difficult to lift and shake heavy glass containers. However, each to his own. Plastic containers are more convenient to carry around and won't crack if dropped accidentally. This

2. 2. Fill the container with water. We do not recommend that you use tap water. Tap water is full of contaminants and impurities which can cause problems with

your readings and the chemical balance of the fertilizer.

A. Fertilizers require purified water. You can buy commercial purified water if you don't have one.

3. Start measuring your nutrients with your digital weighing scale. You can search the Internet to find a calculator for the nutrient concentration if you are unsure about the ratio.

A. The calculator will calculate the proportions or percentages. You should make sure you get the values displayed by the calculator in the smallest unit possible (don't round to the nearest whole number).

4. Before adding salts to the water, make sure you check the pH level. If the pH level is not normal, you can note it. You should not adjust the pH level of the water as the salts can cause it to fluctuate. After you have finished mixing all the ingredients, adjust the water's pH.

5. Slowly pour in the pre-measured salts, one at a. Watch for salts that dissolve well

in water. You can break up any clamps by hand and ensure that the salts are not splashed around when you pour them. This will prevent you from wasting any. You might be surprised at how efficient hydroponics is in growing plants.

6. We are not going to create a concentrated formula because too much of any substance in a hydroponics systems can cause nutrient lock and other diseases in the plants. We are actually diluting salts enough to make them safe for hydroponics.

a. Take a reading of the pH level and take note after adding all the salts to the batch. If necessary, adjust the pH level (see the pH range above). Wait for 2 hours. Allow the solution to rest for at least two hours before you take another pH reading.

Nutrient Ratios for Beginners

These formulae are for one gallon of nutritional solution. You should follow the instructions exactly as fluctuation can cause an imbalance in your system. This is not something you want when you have mature plants.

Formula One
Ratio: 9.5-2.67-11.3
6 grams CA(NO3)2 - 2.99 grams KNO3
- 0.46 grams of K2SO4
1.39 grams KH2PO4
- 2.42g MgSO4 x7H2O
0.40 grams Fe-chelated trace elements

This formula refers to the vegetative or vertical growth states of plants.

Formula Two
Ratio: 8.2-5.9-13.6
- 8 grams CA(NO3)2
- 2.8g of KNO3
- 1.7g of K2SO4
- 1.39g of KH2PO4
- 2.4g MgSO4 x7H2PO
- 0.4% gram Fe chelated trace elements

This formula is used for the flowering and fruiting stages of plants. To ease the transition from vegetative to fruiting stage, use half of each formula.

Formula Three
Fe - 7%

- 2% Mn
- 0.4% Zn
- 1% Cu
- 1.3% B
- 0.06% Mo

This is the formula for the FE-chelated trace element mix

Chapter 9: Choosing The Ideal Plants

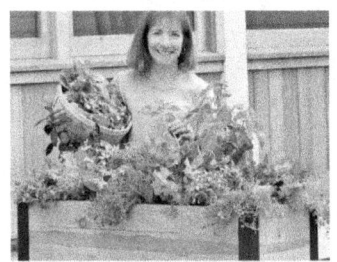

For Your Garden

Now that you have prepared the things that you may need for your garden, the choice of plants is the next consideration. Here we collated a good line up of plants that are happy in containers and are easy to grow. We have classified them into vegetables, herbs, fruits and flowering plants.

The Vegetables Perfect In Containers
Urban gardeners will welcome the idea of having served greens right up their table

from their own garden. It is always an advantage to grow your own veggies, because you can be sure they are of the freshest quality and chemical-free. Here are just some commonly grown vegetables that are perfect for container gardens.

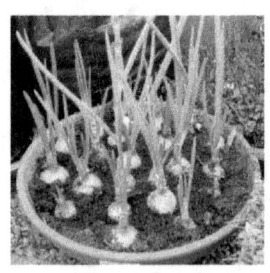

Onions-are one of the easiest veggies to grow in pots. Even for beginners, most varieties of onions will not be difficult to grow and tend to because they thrive in basic conditions. Among the many variety of onions, the green onion are very good for container growing and will thrive even in smaller containers. Harvest them before they are fully mature. To grow them best, the containers should have at least 10 inches of soil depth. Be sure that your pot has good drainage holes and they are a bit elevated from the ground. You can grow them indoors or better yet outdoors where nature takes its course and lest the onion grow as it pleases.

Potatoes are easy to grow in containers. They can grow much basically everywhere, and placing them in a container makes harvesting easy since the tubers is in just one place. It is best to choose good potato seeds. Some variants mature in as much as 70 to 90 days while others may take 120 days before harvest. Any container will do, just make sure that there is enough room to build up the soil as the spuds mature. Growing potatoes require full sun conditions and at least six to eight hours of light exposure. .

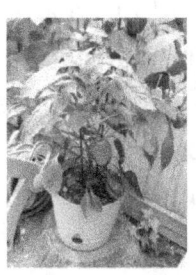

Peppers. Do you like to grow your own peppers in containers? They are also easy and many gardeners find a place for them in their small-scale gardens. If they are in pots, aside from getting fresh peppers for your table, they are also perfect for decorations. They need two important things, that is water and light. It needs five to six hours of direct sunlight and be sure to water it on a daily basis.

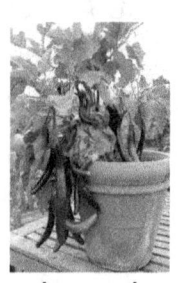

Eggplant is another plant that can be grown easily. In fact other than being a tasty food, they are also ornamental because they bear gorgeous flowers and the special shape of the fruits. For better yield, place your plant in a good container with loamy potting soil. Be sure that your eggplants get enough water to maintain the constant level of moisture perfect for this plant.

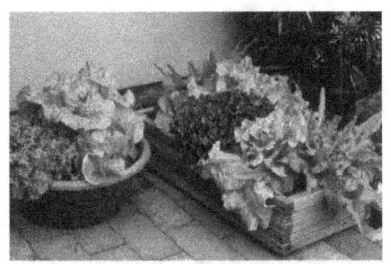

Lettuce is also a thriving plant in a container. It does not need much room. As a cool season crop, the leaves develop best in cool temperatures. Growing your lettuce in a container will help you control weeds as well as pests. And in the moment you need to make a quick salad you just need to get them from the nearby garden. They need consistent supply of moisture and is well-suited to thrive in a container with good drainage holes because they cannot tolerate soggy soil.

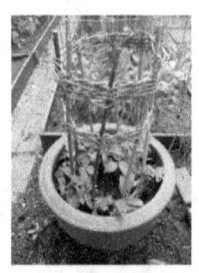

Green beans will grow in warm conditions that containers and pots provide. They are easy to grow and are rich in nutrients when taken as food. Since they adapt well to containers, they are perfect for your container garden. If you choose pole beans, make sure they are given support. They produce all year round and you will find that harvesting them is very easy.

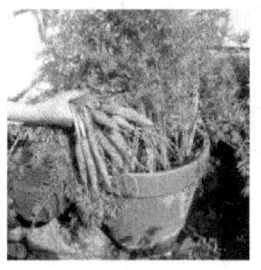

Carrots. The best time to grow them is in early spring or fall. Although some hesitate to plant them in containers because they are a bit difficult to grow, you can try doing so. Just make sure that the soil is lightweight and well-drained. They prefer containers that are deep because they need to develop underneath. Give container grown carrots regular moisture because these gives them optimal growth potential.

Grow Herbs in Containers

Most herbs are perfect container garden plants. They will not occupy much space and will be happy to thrive in any container. These herbs grow best where there is a lot of sunshine. Unlike other plants, herbs do not require a lot of fertilizer at all. They give their best fragrance and flavor devoid of such additives. So lean, unfertilized soil is perfect for them. While most herbs prefer dry conditions, just make sure you water when needed. They will grow best if you provide the soil where there is an excellent drainage and enough space for the roots to grow.

Basil

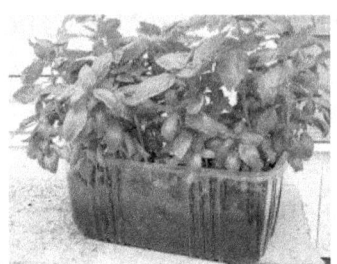

This beloved herb which has its origins in Italy, will grow best where there is plenty of sun and where soil is moist and fertile.

Cilantro

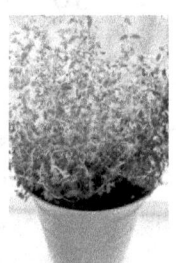

This herb will prefer cooler temperatures so plant it during fall or spring. Also known as coriander, plant it in a container where the container is at least 12 inches deep because of its deep taproot. It will grow best under the sun, although some shade is acceptable for its growth.

Lavender

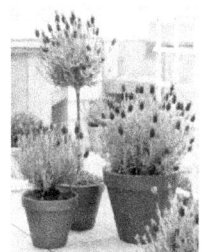

This aromatic herb will later on become a bushy shrub. It will do best under the sun and use a well-drained potting mix to keep it growing. It is a hardy plant that will survive without fertilizer and will not tolerate much water.

Rosemary

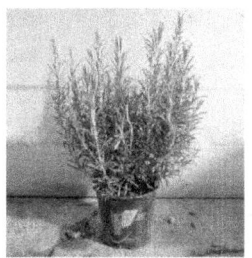

This evergreen shrub, prefers a hot, dry, sunny climate. Because it is drought-tolerant, the key to grow is a dry, quick draining soil. It likes moist but never wet soil mix.

Marjoram

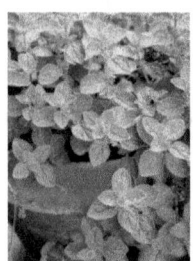

This oregano cousin has a sweeter and milder flavor and aroma. It grows best in full sun and prefers a well-drained soil.

Oregano

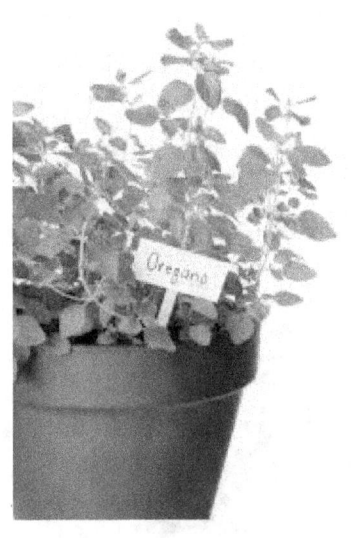

It is an essential ingredient in many Mediterranean dishes. The shrub grows best in plenty of sunshine because the more sun exposure it gets, the more strong the flavors of the leaves.

Mint

This herb is best grown in a pot. It is not picky in terms of soil because it can grow in many types of soil and plenty of sunlight. The best leaves are produced in rich earth, so to make the most of your plant improve the potting mix quality.

This herb comes in plenty of varieties. It does not tolerate overwatering so make sure that it is grown where there is plenty of sunlight and well-drained soil.
Sage

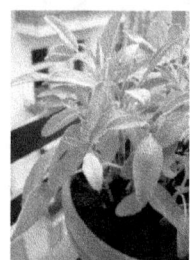

This herb is a favorite for food seasoning particularly in preparing poultry products. You will often find this in many container gardens. This grows best in full sun and well-drained but moist soil mixture.
Growing   Fruits   in   Containers

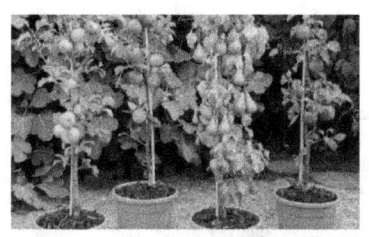

Fruits can also be adapted to grow in pots and containers by those people without adequate space in their homes. The following fruits will fantastically grow in containers and will give you fresh and organic produce when harvest time comes. If you worry about the space they might consume when fully grown, you can also turn to the dwarf varieties of fig, oranges, apples and even strawberries.

Strawberries

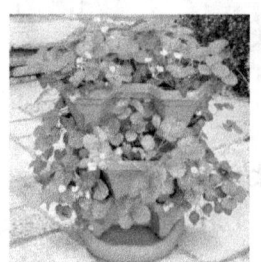

Figs

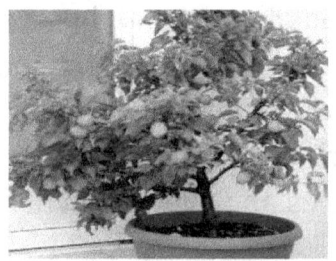

Apples

Lemons

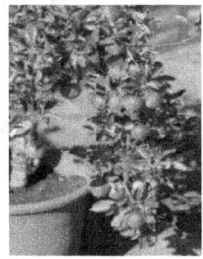 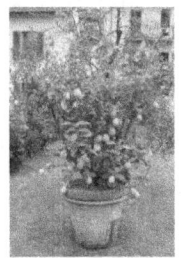

Blueberries

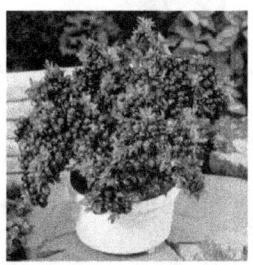

Growing Ornamental and Flowers in Containers

Pretty ornamental and flowering plants will also be perfect for a container garden. Whether you are short on space or have limited time, you can have an attractive set of plants to add scenery to your place.

You can browse through these ornamental plants that will grow their best even in containers. Just remember, this is a very limited selection and you can still have a lot of other flowering plants that you can choose from.

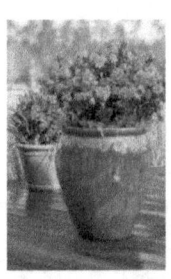

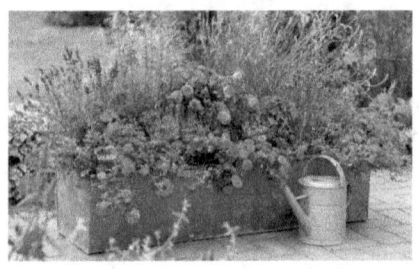

Azaleas will add color to your apartment balcony or veranda. This flowering shrub needs pruning and will thrive in a container which is not well exposed to the sun. If azaleas will begin to have flowers, the blooms will last longer in shadier spots of your mini-garden.

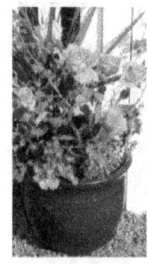

Roses are perfect for any container garden. They grow really quickly and that is the reason why the soil where they are planted will get easily depleted of the nutrients. Not all roses thrive in containers but when they do, they will provide a pleasing sense of freshness in your small space with their beautiful flowers and fragrant aroma.

Chamomile

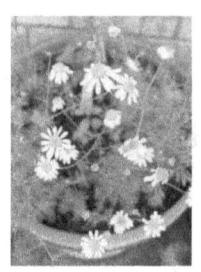

Chamomile. This white-petal flower may appear to look like a daisy but they are different from each other. They are perfect for container gardens and when dried may be used to make a delicious tasting herbal tea.

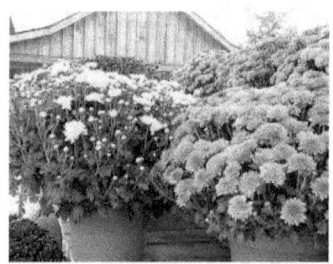

Chrysanthemum flowers, also called mums come in many varieties and colors. They thrive very well in containers and pots and produce very beautiful blooms.

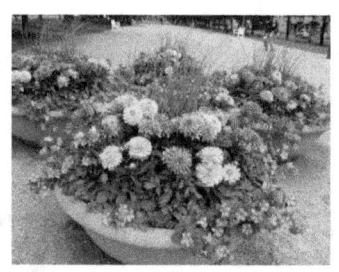

Dahlias do best in flower pots and containers making them a common flowering plant in different varieties that gardeners plant in their gardens. They come in all possible colors except blue.

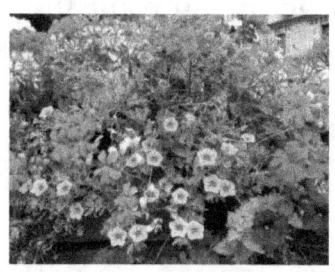

Impatiens. This plant have many species that usually show up in flower beds and are perfect if grown in containers even in shady balconies.

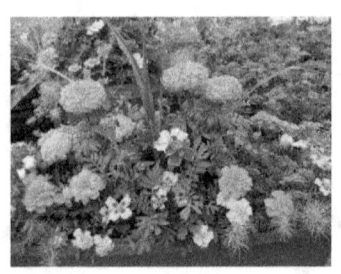

Marigolds are beautiful flowers that you can find in gold, yellow or white and even in mixtures of said colors. They are perfect for the garden because they attract butterflies but repel undesirable insects like mosquitoes due to their strong odor. They are perfect if you plant them beside tomatoes, peppers and potatoes because they prevent the pests from coming closer.

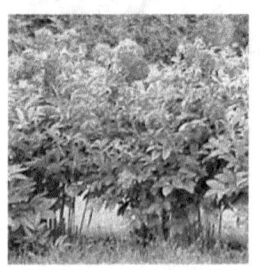

Do not forget peonies because they are not difficult to grow and they produce wonderful, sweet scented flowers. Just make sure that you give their roots a large room because they have deep root systems.

Petunias are classic favorites for container gardening. They come in many colors and will give a colorful display to your garden.

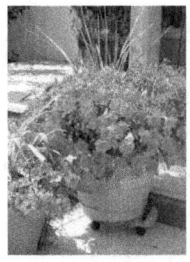

Chapter 10: 7 Reasons Why You Should Get Grow Your Own Vegetables

Do you know there is no doubt that vegetables are great for your health? Even those who don't fancy vegetables would readily admit that they really need to eat them. There are numerous choices in purchasing vegetables e.g., farmers market, supermarket, frozen, and organic. All have their pros and cons, such as availability, price, and freshness.

Everyone will have a varied buying pattern than a large family. Someone with access to a fresh food market or someone with only supermarket access, an occupied person, or time-rich individual.

1. You should know growing vegetables is an affordable therapy!

We all have our goals for our buying habits. Having a vegetable garden is another way of reasoning. It may not be about the food at all. Your vegetable field may become your place of relaxation. (Your moment of calmness in a hectic day). It may be the perfect place to think deeply and plan, or it may just be someplace to hide from the world for a while.

2. It can be your vegetable gym.

Fixing a garden bed, bringing in dirt and fertilizers, and uprooting the weeds are all physical activities that will help your body. Save yourself some gym time, and money, by embracing exercising through digging.

3. You can make it the Kid's time.

Including your children or grandchildren in your green garden will be enjoyable, entertaining, and educational for them. You will need to relax about them being messy, occasionally pulling up the wrong plants, or shaping the rows crookedly. But heh, it's about family fun, not completeness. Give them responsibility for some plants. I remember my son at four, proudly presenting capsicum to us.

Regrettably, it was only tiny, but that didn't matter.

4. It would be perfect for your Kids' health

Do you know their immune systems will considerably benefit from direct access to dirt, resulting in fewer colds and flu? My daughter would gladly be blanketed in dirt from head to toe. It was a lesson for us not to sweat the small stuff, and she has always been a super healthy girl.

5. It would be great for your kids' diet.

You should know children who are part of the vegetable growing process will frequently be better eaters of vegetables. Inspire them to graze in the piece, pick some cherry tomatoes, and baby rocket leaves. Allow them to pick the salad greens for dinner; it would be exciting!

6. Your health.

Hey, it's not all about the kids only! Your health is expected to be greatly improved by planting and growing your vegetables. For all the same reasons that kids benefit, so too will you. These days seem to be confined to stuff in bottles or being prescribed, or things out of your control so much about good health. Growing your vegetables is an essential part of taking control of your bodily and emotional wellbeing.

7. it's perfect for your taste buds.

Do you know packet and tinned foods are mostly taste modified with sugar and salt? Many adults and children don't like the taste of fresh vegetables. Sure, a lettuce leaf is slightly astringent, but you quickly become accustomed to this flavor once you reduce the amount of processed food. Of course, you don't have to eat your homegrown vegetables raw. You can add them to your favorite American, Asian, Italian, or any dish. The health advantages are still there as long as you don't cook them to death.

Chapter 11: How to Make Your Own Energy

Because there are many renewable energy options, homesteading can help you reduce your energy costs. Here are some options:

Wood Fuel

It is a great way to heat your house. A wood stove would be a good option for rural homes. Wood can have a wonderful aroma and feel that can be beneficial to your mind and body. Wood is an affordable alternative to oil and gas for heating your home. Wood can be used as a source of energy and fuel that is renewable and long-lasting. Wood fuel can be used to heat water and cook food. Wood fuel is not enough. You will need other energy sources.

Solar Power

Homesteaders have a great resource of energy in solar power. You can create electricity to power your appliances. To store the sun's energy and provide energy for your home appliances (e.g., a fridge or washing machine), you can install solar panels. Mount the solar panel on your roof, with maximum sunlight exposure. This panel should be kept clear of shadows from trees as they can block sunlight from reaching it.

You can store energy in the daytime to be able to use it consistently at night. This option is great if you live in an area with lots of sun.

Wind Power

Wind turbines can be used to generate electricity. Although this method is noisy, it can still produce electricity for your home appliances. The turbines can be used in conjunction with solar panels if you live in an area that experiences strong winds. To store energy, make sure you hook up a turbine to a battery. It can be difficult for a turbine to be moved in a densely wooded area. To make the turbines move with wind, you should choose a location higher than the trees.

Hydro Power

You can have 24/7 electricity with the power of water. A powerful water stream can generate enough power to provide enough power. This method is useful if you have access to a waterfall. This method is not possible without a waterfall and requires a qualified engineer to set it up. To move the water on a consistent basis, the water flows from one level to another at the bottom of turbine.

This method is the most efficient and cost-effective way to generate energy, compared to any other methods. Water can produce as much as 10 to 100 times the power of solar panels and wind. You can have a constant supply of energy for off-grid living if you use a reliable source. This source can generate consistent energy over a long period of time. The energy can also be stored in batteries for future use. It is important to set up the micro-hydro system in a specific environment. For example, if there is no water source in your backyard it can be very expensive to generate electricity.

Methane

Biogas is also known for natural gas that's produced by rotting organic substances and used as fuel. This is a great way to make biogas from composting plants. This is a cost-effective way to have a home that you can set up on a budget. To get alternative energy for your home, it is a good idea to hire professionals to install any of these options.

Chapter 12: The Best Types Of Fruits

For Home Gardening

Naturally, there are several types of fruits that you can grow in your home garden, but you can't grow them all. Even if you have a small backyard, there are still tons of fruits that you can grow without restrictions. But before planting starts, it's best to put some thoughts into the fruits that grow the best in the climate condition of your state or local area specifically. Fruit trees and bushes can love for as many years as possible, and they require topnotch soil, proper sunlight, and air circulation. Fortunately, some fruit types just go in any garden. These are the best types of fruits to consider having in your garden.

Blueberries are some of the most popular fruits in a backyard homestead; you will likely find them at any backyard garden you visit and for good reasons. Blueberries are very easy to start growing, which is why many new homesteaders often try their hands at growing them as soon as they start fruit gardening. With their attractive shrubs, white flowers, summer fruit, and the red foliage, it is hard not to like blueberries or want them in your garden. Growing blueberries require a soil that is rich and acidic enough to feed them. You may need to do some form of advance work to make the soil acidic enough. The shrubs of a blueberry plant can easily stay alive and produce fruits for many years. To get a good harvest of blueberries at the season-ending, you need to combine two varieties to encourage good pollination. In the colder winter months, grow highbush blueberry varieties like Bluecrop. If you live in a place where the climate is mild, go for the southern highbush rabbiteye blueberries. You may grow your blueberries directly in the soil or in gardening containers. Just ensure that you cover the plants with netting so that they are protected from hungry birds when they start setting fruits. Blueberries usually require full to partial sunlight exposure for survival, and they require a soil mix that is incredibly rich, acidic, mildly or eagerly moist, and well-draining.

Strawberries that are freshly picked from the farm are usually worth the effort that you put into growing them. You have three options for your strawberry plants:

June bearing which is great for planting in June as a large crop but has a shorter fruiting season;

Everbearing, which produces three to four smaller harvests each season

Day-neutral, which continuously produces small batches of strawberries throughout the whole growing system.

Generally, strawberries spread through runners. But if you want to have great production, your runners shouldn't be more than a few plants – prune the remaining plants. Also, be sure to pinch away the blossoms in your first planting season to prevent it from setting fruit. This is a way to help it channel its energy towards building a well-protected and healthy root season. After the first season, the production in the next season will increase to a significant extent. Finally, make sure you change or swap out your strawberry plant every 3 to 5 years Or, at the very least, make sure that you rejuvenate the plants in this timeframe. Strawberries need full sunlight exposure, and the soil for planting should be very rich, a little acidic, mildly moist or set, and be well-draining.

Apples are difficult to grow than most crops usually, but many homesteaders still want to have them in their garden. A basic idea of fruit gardening will tell you that apple trees are often affected by different pest and disease problems. New apple cultivars may be grown to be hardy. Still, you also need to protect them in your own ways, by covering, spraying, and other protection techniques that should be incorporated swiftly, specifically as soon as planting starts. Apple plants also tend to require a lot of pruning, which is another reason why homesteaders are wary of growing apples. To grow apple, you need two apple tree varieties to achieve pollination. Choose trees with several varieties that are grafted into a trunk, or go for a columnar tree, which can be homegrown in your containers. If you have limited space, you can plant the dwarf apple varieties. Pruning and thinning is essential for promoting good health and disease prevention in your plants. So, ensure they are a part of your routine when you are caring for your fruit garden. Apples grow best under full sun exposure, and you want the soil to be rich, mildly moisture as well as have poor well-drawn.

Raspberries and blackberries are favorites among homesteaders. For years, they have always been a part of most homegrown fruit gardens. But older varieties of raspberries and blackberries usually grow to be rambunctious plants, which means they quickly spread around the garden and become covered in thorns to the point that harvesting becomes a significantly difficult and painful task. Newer varieties are much better because they behave better, and they grow to be thornless. Moreover, the best idea is to plant a mix of the early, mid-season, and late-season raspberry and blueberry varieties as this helps to extend your harvest for many more weeks. These plants need you to prune them annually to keep them protected and productive, but this task is usually quite easy. The aim of pruning is to thin out the plant significantly to allow sunlight and air to reach every part of the plants. This promotes growth and helps with disease and pest control. In USDA growing zones, you will need 5 to 8 raspberry and blackberry for your backyard farm. The ideal sun exposure for these fruits' ranges from full sun to partial shade.

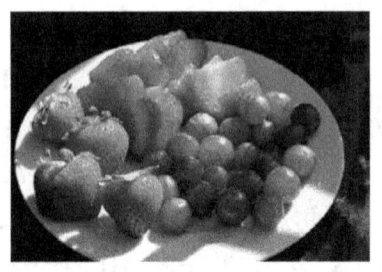

Grapes are another incredible fruit that should be a part of any home garden. Normally, grapevines are easy and straight forward to grow. Still, competition often comes from birds and other farm animals who want to have a taste of your grapes. Plus, you need to build support – sort of like a trellis – for grapes to grow on. Also, there are different instructions on the best way to prune grapes. Still, most gardeners can grow them successfully without using an aggressive pruning approach. Before you plant your grapevine, make sure you check with the local extension office in your local area to get valuable information on the best grape varieties to grow. And make sure you check whether the variety that is recommended to you is good for winemaking or eating. Most eatable grape varieties need to be located in a sunny part of the garden with rich soil, good drainage, and sufficient air circulation to prevent possible disease attacks. The right exposure for grapes generally is full sun.

Cherries are quite easy to grow, care for, and maintain. Unlike many fruits, they require little pruning sessions and very rarely suffer from pests or disease attack. To cross-pollinate, cherries must have two trees. Otherwise, you will need to plant one tree with two different grape varieties on it. Moreover, if you are focusing on just spur baking cherries, you can get away with planting just one tree. The best time to prune cherry trees is during the winter while it is inactive. Then, you should fertilize and add organic matter in early spring. Since cherry trees are not known to be drought-tolerant, ensure that you water them at least weekly in the hot months and let the rainfall take care of them during fall. Cherries need full sun exposure to grow and mature as you want.

Peaches tend to have very small trees that will fit right in any backyard farm, no matter the size. When peaches start ripening, their sweetness can be smelled from yards away. Additionally, one of the benefits of growing peaches yourself is that you get to enjoy the freshness straight from the source, instead of the stale and potentially-damaged options that are sold at the supermarket. To keep the branches of your peaches' tree productive and manageable, you will need to do some pruning from time to time. Thinning young peaches tree helps them produce small-sized crops of large peaches, instead of heavy crops of tiny ones. Peaches require full sun exposure every day to get all the nutrients they need.

Figs are another fruit that can be grown directly in the ground or in a gardening container. They are generally pest-free and are known to require very little pruning. There are different fig varieties that you can get to plant in your garden, and many of them are known to be quite hardy. In fact, some of the newest varieties are even hardier than the rest. If you want to grow your figs in a gardening container so that you can keep it indoors during winter, make sure the container is as small as possible. The less space between the roots, the smaller the treetop will remain. Plus, a small container is much easier to move around than a big one. And regardless of the size of the container, you will still get enough fig fruit to feast on with your family. Figs need full sun to partial shade sun exposure to grow in the right condition. Plus, the soil mix for growing figs should be rich with organic matter, moist, and loosely-draining.

Melons are the go-to fruit for the new homesteader that isn't quite ready for the commitment required by fruit trees, bushes, and shrubs. This is because they can be easily grown in containers or in the garden if it is what you wish. Melons require a lot of sun exposure and warmth as part of their growing condition. They also require ample spacing, as they usually grow on vines, which can easily grow up to 20 feet and more. You may be able to grow your melons on a trellis, but only if you purchase a variety with small-sized fruits. Watermelon varieties often become so heavy that they end up dropping off the plant. Start planting your melon right after the final frost, and make sure you keep them watered regularly to establish their growth. Once the fruits start to appear, you can ease off on watering. Melons, regardless of their varieties, require a full sun exposure to grow healthily. Additionally, the planting soil must be loamy, well-endowed with nutrients, and well-drained.

Companion Planting

Companion planting is a method of planting that you should really consider as you start to expand your gardening. This method of planting goes beyond the idea that some plants can benefit others when they are planted in proximity to each other. Companion planting is the planting of two or more crops of the same species together to control pests better and increase the yield. Although companion planting is mostly used for vegetables by many farmers, it also applies to fruits, and it is something you should consider using with your backyard garden. Many fruits grow amazingly well when they are planted with other crops. Below is a list of some fruits that should be in your garden and suitable companion plants:

- Blackberries – strawberries, dewberries
- Cucumber – peas, beans
- Figs – mustards, dandelions
- Grapes – blackberries, peas
- Apricot – chives, leeks
- Melon – pigweed, chamomile
- Peach – Basil
- Raspberries – tansy
- Sweet corn – pumpkin, squash
- Strawberries – onions, lettuce
- Tomatoes – pepper, cabbage

Of course, many other fruits can be grown alongside their companion plants. Companion planting is a really effective method that new gardeners can use to minimize the risks of pest invasion on their new farms.

Now that you know the exact types of fruits that you want in your backyard garden, let's get to the part where you actually plan and plant the fruits.

Chapter 13: Maximizing Your Space

Maximizing the space of your mini farm can be done in several ways. Sometimes, all it takes is an open mind and a fearless imagination to think of solutions to space problems, and help your farm expand without necessarily purchasing more land to work on.

Ideas for the Innovative Urban Mini Farmer

Here are three fun and practical ideas to help you maximize your space and harvest!

Companion Planting for Maximized Plot Space

1. Learn all about Companion planting and apply it to your gardens, both indoors and out! Companion planting teaches all gardeners that some crops play well with others and actually encourage each other's growth, while others should not be anywhere near one another. By knowing which plants are friendly together, you can

use just one garden plot for three or even five different plants!

Vertical Gardening for Wall and Ceiling Gardens

2. Vertical gardening is the answer for tight spaced mini farms. If you can't spread your pots on the ground, don't despair! Look for ways to scale your pots upwards. Invest in cheap shoe racks and convert them into plant racks, add hooks to the ceilings, and make use of terrace beams for crawling crops. You can even attach shelves along the top quarter of your walls and store pots there.

Aquaponics: Hitting Fish and Herbs with One Stone!

3. If you love fish but don't have enough space for a wide fish pond, then you should learn all about aquaponics. Aquaponics is the art of growing herbs, and small vegetables in the same water tank used to raise fish. By learning and applying the techniques of aquaponics, you will be able to harvest both fresh fish and herbs!

Chapter 14: The Need For Community

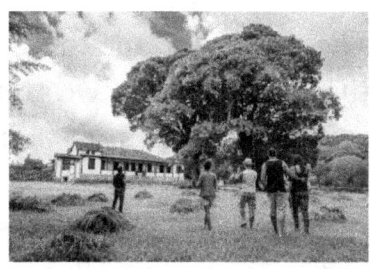

Whether you live completely off the grid or you have a more urban backyard homestead, the key to successful, self-sufficient living lies in your community. Being involved with people who share similar opinions will result in tons of new lessons learned, friendships built, and, most importantly, easy adjustment to your new lifestyle.

By reaching out to your community you will find many fellow homesteaders who are willing to teach, share, and give you a helping hand. Just think about having someone to tell you that the mulch you were planning on adding could potentially kill your plants due to chemical release. Or having a friend you can exchange your goods with? Or swapping extra zucchini for a bag of plums that are yet to mature can be a true jackpot. Depending on your location, there are many ways in which you can get involved with a community.

Get in Touch – Locally

You cannot possibly be the only homesteader in your area. Ask around and get in touch with like-minded people. You can do this by attending classes or attending the farmer's market. Joining a local group will be of huge help, especially if you are just starting out. If you don't know where to start, you can do a local search online (think Facebook) or even try Craigslist. You can also ask your local library to point you in the right direction.

Pinterest

Okay, this is not exactly a social platform where you can meet new people, but searching for off-grid projects, farms, and homesteads can bring valuable information your way. Not only can you get inspired by the things that you care about, you will also find many new homesteading blogs and forums where you can get in touch with people who live sustainably.

Blogs and Forums

If your area is so rural that you cannot afford trips to your library or farmer's market, you can always try to find a community online. Searching for homesteading blogs and forums is a great way to start. Find a topic you are interested in (like raised-bed gardening or milking a goat), and do some digging. Check the comment section to find more people to connect with.

Facebook

Facebook is the obvious choice when searching for an online community. There are many established homesteading groups there, so join some and connect with similar folks. Who knows, you may even find some that live close by!

Try It Yourself

Cannot find a local farming community? Build one yourself! Make business cards and hand contact info wherever you can – at the farmer's market, library, local extension office. Hand out flyers and hold events. Hold a bonfire where you can share some of your rich harvest. Reach out to people and find a like-minded bunch. It will be a lot easier if you connect to a group, both geographically and ideologically.

Chapter 15: How To Build A New Flower Bed For All Your Favorite Blooms

A flower bed gives you a place to plant colorful annuals and perennials that can fill your yard with beauty. And flowers, of course, are essential for butterflies and other pollinators, so creating more space for blooming plants will help roll out the welcome mat for these beneficial creatures. Like a blank canvas, a new flower bed offers you the chance to get creative and fill it with whatever you can imagine (quilt garden, anyone?). The options are nearly endless, but first comes the actual building part. This might seem like a daunting project, but with a little planning, preparation, and sweat equity, you'll soon be enjoying a more beautiful, flower-filled garden.

How to Prepare a Flower Bed

When you're starting from scratch, there are a few things to consider first. Here are the questions you need to answer:

Where will it go?

Anywhere from a corner of the backyard to your front entryway can make a great spot for a flower bed. You can place one along a deck or porch, underneath a tree, or around a garden feature like a pond, for example. If you plant near a driveway or along a curb, be sure to consider traffic safety when it comes to plant height, and if you live where it will get icy in the winter, keep in mind salt spray, which can kill plants.

How much sunlight will the bed get?

Many popular bedding plants like annual flowers require full sun, which means a minimum of six hours of direct sunlight each day. You can certainly choose a spot in part-sun or even a mostly shady area, but you'll be a bit more limited in what flowers will grow there.

What's the soil like?

Most flowering annuals and perennials appreciate a loamy soil with plenty of compost added to it. Make sure to rake away rocks or other debris from the site, break up any large clods of dirt, and add compost to enrich the bed and encourage healthy plant growth. It's also a good idea to do a soil test to find out if you should add any nutrients your plants will need to look their best.

Flower Bed Ideas and Designs

Once you've chosen a site, it's time for the fun part: Flower bed design. Here are some ideas to spark your imagination.

Looking to a make a statement in front of the house? Wrap a small flower bed around your mailbox, line your front walkway, add color underneath a tree, or surround the bases of the front porch risers.

Get geometric with a perfectly square, rectangular, circular, or even triangular bed.

Focus on tall or dense plants to help block unattractive backyard features such as air conditioners, trash cans, swimming pool heaters, or storage sheds.

Removing Grass and Building the Flower Bed

Unless you've got an already bare patch of earth, you'll need to remove the turf before planting your flowers. After marking the outline of your new flower bed with spray paint or white flour, there are two basic ways to remove the grass on the inside of your lines.

Dig up existing grass.

Digging out the grass can be hard work. Use a shovel to remove a section of grass from the center of your planned bed, then continue to remove turf by wedging the shovel (a hoe also works) under the edges of the grass. Then lift and peel the sod away. Once you have removed the grass, you can prepare the soil for planting.

Make a flower bed without digging.

Removing grass without digging is the lengthy-but-easy method. Simply cover the entire area of your future flower bed with several overlapping sheets of newspaper. Layer the paper at least six pages deep, then cover the newspaper with several inches of rich soil or compost. Water well. Over the next few months, the buried grass will die, and the newspaper will decompose while adding nutrients to the soil. For best results, keep the area covered for up to a year before planting.

Once the turf has been removed, outline the area with some landscape edging made of plastic, stone, brick, or wood. Some quirky materials you can use for edging include glass bottles, large seashells, or decorative metal fencing.

Build a raised flower bed.

There are a few ways to do this. You can use wood boards cut to the desired length. This lets you build whatever shape or size you desire. But if you prefer the simplest solution, there are raised flower bed kits that supply everything you need, and easily snap together with no need for sawing or hammering. Most kits create fairly small squares or rectangles.

If you're going to build your raised flower bed on top of existing grass, first cover the turf with a few sheets of newspaper, then top the paper with good-quality planting mix, and finish off with a layer of compost. If you want to build on top of concrete or another hard surface, you'll first need a protective bottom layer of plywood, landscape fabric, or heavy plastic sheeting to keep soil from slowly spreading out of the raised bed and discoloring the concrete.

Flower Bed Plants

You designed your flower bed, you removed the grass, you prepared the soil, and you edged your soon-to-be-planted site. Now it's time to plant! You'll want to choose varieties that do well in your climate, of course, and are suited to your site's exposure to sunlight. But beyond that, the best flowers are the ones you love the most.

Low-growing annuals such as sweet alyssum, lobelia, and impatiens work well as front-of-the-border plants.

Add zing in the front of the house with a colorful mixture of varied-height beauties like zinnias, snapdragons, or marigolds.

Tall flowers, including sunflowers, hollyhocks, and cosmos, can be especially inviting when flanking the steps to your front porch or along a property fence.

Raised flower bed planting ideas include a center row of tall and medium-height blooms with a border of cascading flowers like bacopa, ivy geranium, moss rose, or calibrachoa.

Other ideas include a garden of single-color flowers, a patriotic mix of red-white-and-blue blooms, a pastel flower bed, or a "moon garden" planted entirely in white flowers

What Supplies Are Needed for an Outdoor Flower Garden

Bed Development

Developing the bed involves marking out the outline of your bed and cutting it. While you may choose to "free-hand" it, a well-marked bed allows you to make the curves and corners exactly where you need them, instead of guessing. The bed should go at least 2 feet past where you'll place the end planting holes. Mark the bed outline with rope or a garden hose and then cut it with a D-handled straight hoe or straight edger. Once you've edged out the outline of your bed, you can move onto soil prep.

Soil Preparation

Soil preparation is the first step in creating a garden that will be functional as well as productive. Preparation involves amending and tilling the soil, making it rich, loose and right for your flowers or ornamental plants. The two main supplies: a tiller and rich, organic compost. Till the plot to a workable 12 inches or so and till the bed 2 feet past where your last plants will be on the ends. Follow with tilling a thick layer of compost about 6 to 10 inches into the top of the soil. Your end result is loose soil, rich in organic matter that drains well and provides a smooth enough soil for the roots of your plants to grow in and take nutrients from. If you are tilling a small bed or are up for some heavy labor, you can use a long-handled garden cultivator instead of a powered tiller. After tilling, rake the soil using a long-handled garden rake so that it's level and smooth. If you'll be filling the whole bed with flowers and ornamental plants, you can fertilize the soil with a broadcast spreader and all-purpose or starter fertilizer, generally at a rate of 2 cups per 100 feet of garden bed. All fertilizers vary, so read the instructions for exact application rates.

Planting Time Supplies

Planting's the fun part -- at least for most people. You'll need a couple of supplies for planting, and the list could change depending on if you're planting seeds, bulbs or plants in pots from the garden center. For plants in pots less than 1 quart, a gardening trowel will do the trick. For pots larger than 1 gallon, you'll need a narrow shovel to dig the planting holes. You can use a trowel or bulb planter for bulbs, while seeds typically require nothing more than your fingers. Once the plants are in the ground, water them thoroughly and then apply 3 to 4 inches of organic mulch around them and over the bed. Organic mulch, such as untreated wood chips, regulates the soil temperature and moisture.

Care Supplies

Once your flowers are blooming, you'll need to keep a few tools handy to keep them looking their best. A pair of sharp, scissor-cut pruners work well for deadheading spent blooms and cutting stalks to the ground in fall or early spring. Specialty handheld weeding tools will help you dig out weeds around your plants. Soaker or drip hoses to lay at the base of your flowers will help you water correctly: deeply and over the roots.

Extras

While these tools may not be necessities, they can help you -- and your body -- out along the way. Gardening gloves will help protect your hands from thorny plants and blisters from holding gardening tools. A foam knee mat may sound superfluous, but it can help prevent sore, cracked and aching knees at the end of a long day of planting or weeding. A wheelbarrow or yard cart is useful for carrying tools or flower pots from the shed to your bed and can greatly ease tension on your lower back. Last but not least: a sun hat of some sort. Get one that suits your style -- they come in all shapes and sizes from the stylish to the downright crazy.

Pots and Containers

The age and planting method of the flower determine what type of container to use. Small seedling pots, cell-packs or flats provide a suitable growing container for planting seeds indoors for later outdoor transplanting. Plants to remain potted require a pot large enough to hold the mature flower. An 8- to 12-inch-diameter pot usually suffices. Pots and containers need drainage holes in the bottom so water doesn't collect inside the pots. Placing drip trays to catch the draining water under indoor flower pots prevents spills.

Soil

Potting soil mixtures can contain peat, compost, vermiculite, perlite and soil. The amount of each material depends on the type of potting soil. Soilless mixes provide a sterile and well-draining choice for both seedlings and mature flowers. Mixes containing soil only work well for mature plants. A potting mix may already contain fertilizers, but those formulated for planting seeds usually come unfertilized.

Planting Amendments

Amendments, such as compost and fertilizer, help improve the soil quality in garden beds. Compost improves the quality of the soil, aids proper moisture retention and provides trace nutrients. A preplanting or "start fertilizer" application before or right at planting provides the nutrients the flowers need to produce a healthy root system and lush foliage growth. Most beds require a second fertilization at midseason to provide the nutrients for continued bloom.

Tools

Potted flowers require few tools. A narrow trowel helps dig planting holes to the correct depth in larger pots, but isn't necessary for small pots or seed starting. A hoe helps break up soil clods in garden beds and proves useful for cultivating and preventing weeds between the flowers once they are planted. Tall flowers with weak stems, such as peonies, may require stakes installed at planting to help support the flowers.

Mulching

Mulching improves the moisture level in the soil of outdoor beds. Organic mulches like bark nuggets, pine straw and wood chips provide an attractive mulch option for ornamental beds. Inorganic mulches, like plastic or landscape fabric, also prevent most weeds from growing when installed under organic mulch. Plastic and fabric mulch need to be applied to the bed prior to planting; organic mulches are applied after the flowers are planted.

Essential Garden Tools Every Gardener Should Own

Wheelbarrow

We have a selection of galvanised and hard plastic wheelbarrows available. A good barrow is strong yet light enough to easily transport when full. Also, why not try one of these water carrying bags for wheelbarrows, they are the only way to transport water in a barrow without spilling it. Wheelbarrow – Hard plastic and 100 Litre capacity

solid Oak Dibber for planting seeds and seedlings 9. Dibber Dibbers are useful for making planting holes for seeds, bulbs and seedlings. We have a nice selection of oak timber dibbers as well as some stainless steel ones, the timber ones have calibrated rings to indicate depth and take the guesswork out of planting.

Digging Spade

A decent digging spade is always needed in the garden, in my opinion the best one to use is a stainless steel type. Regular spades easily rust and the soil tends to stick to them whereas a good stainless steel spade stays smooth making digging that much easier

. Garden Trowel

Hand tools like garden trowels and hand forks are some of the most used gardening tools, so the best trowel should have a comfortable handle with a well fitted blade that won't come loose after time. This transplanting trowel from Burgon & Ball has a comfortable ash timber handle with a stainless steel blade with planting depths etched into the face.

. Fork Hoe

Chillington Tools (the crocodile range), need no introduction on this site, they are the cornerstone of our garden tools list. Chillington hoes all have their digging blades at a right angle to the handle, in the traditional 'Mattock' style, this gives better leverage making digging alot easier.

Garden Knife

A small knife is often needed in the garden for cutting string, sticks and flowers, trimming fruit and vegetable plants and many other jobs. It's a good habit to carry one in your pocket or garden trug. Opinel knives have a very sharp blade that folds into the wooden handle. These knives were ranked in the top 100 most beautiful products in the world by the Victoria and Albert Museum

Garden Secateurs

Any garden needs constant maintenance and a good garden secateurs is an invaluable tool to have for any pruning jobs. The secateurs we recommend is the Classic Felco no4, they are affordable bypass secateurs that will last a lifetime.

Heavy Duty Hoe

. This time it is the heavy duty garden hoe. This hoe is ideal for breaking new ground and will do so much easier than a spade or shovel. Like the fork hoe, it's blade is set at a right angle to the handle allowing the lever action to minimise effort required.

Golden Gark

The Golden Gark is a multipurpose garden maintenance tool, it is a rake, shovel and soil sift in one. This lightweight tool is ideal for clearing up weeds or fallen autumn leaves and much more.

. Oscillating Hoe

This is another tool that needs no introduction on this site, the oscillating hoe is a long handled garden hoe with a swivel head. The long handle enables you to hoe an entire raised bed from the same position and the swivel action head cuts on both the puch and the pull stroke sharpening itself as it goes.

Chapter 16: How To Learn About Homesteading:

If you're making the shift from gardening to homesteading, there are a number of valuable ways to educate yourself and add to your skillset. Plus, they're fun, which makes learning any new skill-less fearful and more exciting.

Read books and watch videos. I can't tell you how much I've learned about homesteading by simply watching a video or reading a book. As we got into raising goats, we'd be outside with new clippers looking at a YouTube video about how to trim their hooves. And my bookshelf is now filled with books and magazines on natural chicken-raising, food-growing, and setting up a home apothecary. It all seems difficult until you've seen it done or had it explained to you.

Cultivate like-minded friendships. Some of my best friends are people I can call in a pinch when we're having trouble with goat birthing (thanks, Chris M.!), and others I've met along the way through social media, buying supplies at the feed store, or when purchasing an animal from them. Look for local homesteading/chicken keeping/apiary groups and join their meet-ups, and be open to high-quality Facebook groups on the homesteading topic of your interest.

Attend natural living, wellness, and earth fairs. We just attended one with a friend a couple of weeks ago, in fact. We sat in on seminars about cultivating mushrooms, browsed the bookstore and met authors, chatted with vendors, and met some new friends. Well worth the price of admission.

The Great Benefits of Homesteading

Homesteading is humbling:

As a homesteader, one quickly realizes just how small one is and how finite life is. For any homesteader, mistakes will be overwhelming. Animals will die. Crops will be ruined. Structures fall down. Plans fall through. It's humbling to attempt and tame a piece of this Earth, only to have it implode time after time. Which – hear me now – it will. The chickens may be eaten by an owl or the cow may stick her food in the milk bucket – but regardless of the failings that will inevitable come, homesteading continues. So while it may be an extremely humbling road to wander down, the perseverance bred through the humbling failures is not to be missed. It's character building, don't you think? To fail, recognize one's inability to control life, pray for grace, and then continue on.

Homesteading builds a strong work ethic:
Work ethic is something strongly missing in our culture, don't you think? I've recently been rereading Farmer Boy and am taken back by the amount of work that was expected of children. At the ripe 'ol age of six? seven? they're milking cows. Feeding animals. Training oxen. Cooking supper alongside their Mom. Kids are CAPABLE and thrive in such environments. While I'm thankful that our lifestyle no longer requires such labor from our

children, it's important that the idea of building up ourselves (and our children) with strong work ethics isn't thrown out with the bathwater.

If anything will build up a solid work ethic, it's the responsibility that comes with growing food so that our family can EAT (ya. kinda important.) or raising animals that are reliant on us, day after day, for their survival.

The instant negativity associated with laziness in instantly felt on the homestead. The best way to breed it out is to slather it in work!

Homesteading tastes good!:

Many of y'all are chicken owners – you know the beautiful, orange, perky yolks that come from a well-loved and healthy hen. The taste is indistinguishable. I've ever surprised (why? I don't know) at the incredibly depth of difference of homegrown food to conventional food. Again, I think it's important to note: I'm very thankful that my survival is not dependent on my own ability to produce food. I think it's important and progressive that we have such food available to us year-round. But that being said, a lot of it just ain't good.

Ever tasted an out-of-season-picked-green-raspberry? It's like a flavorless gob of nastiness.

Even my hard to convince husband was undoubtedly convinced at our last dinner date out – he ordered the roast chicken. "Well, it sure isn't like our Rainbow Rangers. It's sort of flat tasting and squishy." (You can read more about meat chickens here.) I felt the same about my steak, which was cooked and flavored beautifully, but still fell incredibly short of the grass-fed local meat we're used to. We spent the rest of the dinner planning how we could grow MORE of these things ourselves if for no other reason than the taste!

We're foodies. We like food that tastes the best.

And homegrown food tastes the best – fresh tomatoes from the summer garden, pastured eggs, homemade butter, fresh salsa, you name it. And I guarantee you it tastes better when you've grown it yourself.

I'd be hard pressed to find anyone who would disagree.

Homesteading breeds appreciation:

Back to those fresh tomatoes. Remember the first one you ate out of your garden last year? I bet you do. Because before you could taste that first tomato, you had to put in months of work planting seeds, caring for tender seedlings, planning the proper time to plant them out, protecting them from harsh weather, nurturing them as they grew and blossomed, trellising them as they became heavy with fruit, and patiently waiting for them finally ripen. And when that first delicious orb is removed from the vine, it's hard to not be brought to tears. I guarantee you that after hand milking a cow, you'll never look at a gallon of milk the same way, and the same goes for millions of tasks on the homestead.

Nothing breeds appreciation like knowing the hard work that went into providing our family with something.

I think this also correlates very closely with the homesteading mantra: "Use it up, wear it out, make it do, or do without". When the items that one grows or produces holds such extreme value, they tend to be treated far better and made to last, as well as utilized to their maximum. It's hard to find homesteaders that are wasteful – they appreciate the value of everything (even if it's garden scraps or manure for the compost pile).

Homesteading adds a new value to meat:

If you've ever grown your own your own meat, you know two things: 1. Meat takes an incredible amount of energy (ie: feedstuff) to raise and 2. Taking the life of the animal you are raising for meat is hard. Let's start with the first point – the amount of energy it takes to raise meat. Whether this be in the form of grass or grain, the amount it takes to raise the mean is quite astounding. Because of this, we've found that the amount of meat that we eat has been greatly affected. We don't eat it at every meal. We don't even eat it every day. Limited resources of energy in the form of feed means limited amount of meat. Because vegetables and eggs can be grown here with such fewer resources than meat, that's a huge portion of what we eat. They are easier, cheaper, and require less energy to produce. Not something one really has to think about when purchasing meat from the store, but for a homestead, it's a really important equation to consider.

Taking the life of our meat animals also adds a new value to eating this protein. As was the case with our rabbits and our chickens, it was with great sadness and a profound appreciation that we slaughtered and butchered them for our consumption. It's not something to be taken lightly and when we've actually had to do the raising, killing, and processing of the animals ourselves we've found the meat to be far more valuable to us.

Homesteading develops a truer sense of gender roles:

We hold to a Biblical view and belief of gender roles and life on the homestead has proven those gender roles to be so true and necessary. Stuart is so strong and capable of many of the manual labor tasks that I am physically incapable of. I wish I was buffer – but I ain't. And so it goes. While nursing Owen, catering to nap schedules, preserving food, and preparing meals, I find myself naturally more drawn to work in the home (or that which can be done in the garden or in the coop with the children). While this isn't always the case (as I often lend Stuart a hand with big projects, bucking hay, or building fence) it's given me a new appreciation for my role as a Christian woman and as a wife, helpmeet, and mother.

I see great value in the chores that not only keep this homesteading running but also are of great service to this family.

Life on the homestead has caused me to see how these roles became so defined in times past — I picture a woman with a child on each hip, a giant white apron smeared with kitchen projects, and a few chickens following her around the yard. It's a beautiful thing and in no way less meaningful or important. All work on the homestead is extremely valuable and all of it is required to keep it running smoothly. Someone's gotta milk. Someone's gotta cook biscuits for breakfast. And someone's gotta butcher the animals.

Homesteading increases knowledge:
Like anything you commit time and energy to, naturally, knowledge is gained on the subject matter. Running a homestead has been no different. We've learned about everything from native grasses, to feed conversions, to heritage breeds, to the patterns and cycles of the honey bee, to milking a dairy cow, to fencing options, to soil assessments, to composting, to pollination, to cheese making, to water and energy usage, to first aid, to gutting a chicken, and everything in between.

Homesteading breeds dreams:

As of yet, we've never found that nirvana of perfection with our homestead. We're always looking forward to what we can do better, more efficiently, and with improved results. Once we are successful with one project, it's time to expand the operation and dream bigger!

I love to dream. It's one of my favorite past times. It keeps us working and hopeful for what is to come!

While these great benefits of homesteading may not be true for every homesteader, we've found them to be very true to ours. At the risk of sounding cliche, homesteading has developed our character and grown us into better people of faith. We rely on the Lord for all the happenings every day on the homestead and are so thankful for every day that we get to continue on this journey with our land and our animals.

It's not a perfect life, and it's not for everyone, but it is pretty dang rad. If you ask me.

Chapter 17: Save And Generate Your Own Energy

Since there are lots of choices for you, but you need to compare their costs to pick a one best for you. The electricity produced through these sources will be really cheap as compared to the electricity obtained from the national grid. Following are some approximate prices for the equipment (only material). This table has no installation charges, so add these charges in this cost to get an accurate estimate.

Source to Produce Electricity	Total Power	Total Cost
Solar Panel	1 KW	$6,000
Dual Axis Tracker		$6,250
Wind Generator with a 50 foot tower	1 KW	$3,700
Batteries for the reserve of one		$8,000

day		
Inverter or charger	4 KW	$3,000
Total cost		$26,950
Note: It is an estimated cost, but it may vary widely based on the various regions.		

If you expected to get the sunlight and air for almost eight hours, then you can use a solar panel and wind generator to produce electricity. You can produce almost 487 kW-hour electricity in a month with your new resources.

Electrical Inverter

The inverters or charger is available with almost a 20-year lifespan to produce almost 116,880 kW-hours electricity. The cost of the electricity can be $0.23 per kW-hour.

Backup Generator

You can recharge the batteries with the help of gasoline to get almost 3.5 kW-hour electricity after burning a gallon of fuel. The fuel cost will be almost $1.00 per kW and in this way, you can save almost 40% cost of the energy.

Conclusion

Thank you again for downloading this book!

I hope this book was able to help you to find all the ways by using which you can opt for modern homestead techniques. In the present world, where price of everything is going up and up, it becomes very difficult for a mediocre family to live a perfect life with each and every expense to get fulfilled. But, even in difficult situations, you cannot only save the extra money you have but you can also become able to cut down your expenses by investing a little amount of money in homesteading. This process does not requires a lot of money to be spent but yes, you are definitely required to give some of your extra time to it. Dedication and proper working upon the techniques of homesteading will help you out in making it so perfect and successful in all aspects.

The next step is to act upon all the pieces of advice and tips which I have added in this book for you. By carefully acting upon all the tips of this book, you will definitely help yourself in saving your money along with getting extravagant benefits from your own backyard farm without any problem.

www.ingramcontent.com/pod-product-compliance
Lightning Source LLC
Chambersburg PA
CBHW071825080526
44589CB00012B/923